A Lion in the House

A Lion in the House

FIVE FAMILIES. SIX YEARS.
TRUE STORIES FROM THE WAR ON CANCER

The Companion Volume
to the Award-winning
PBS Documentary
by Steven Bognar & Julia Reichert

Edited by Margaret A. McGurk

ORANGE FRAZER PRESS
Wilmington, Ohio

ISBN: 1-933197-20-X

Copyright © 2006 by A Lion In The House, LLC

No part of this publication may be reproduced in any form or by any means, electronic or mechanical, including any information storage and retrieval systems, without permission from the publisher, except by reviewers who may wish to quote briefly.

Orange Frazer Press, Inc.
P.O. Box 214
Wilmington, OH 45177
800-852-9332
www.orangefrazer.com

Cover design: Jeff Fulwiler

Book design: Chad DeBoard and Jeff Fulwiler

Project Coordinator: Melissa Godoy

Chapter 8 compiled by Karen Durgans

Production Assistance: Dan Misch, Dylan Hay

Copy Editors: Jeanette Murray, Rebecca Caires

Proofreaders: Melissa Godoy, Karen Durgans, Lee Huntington, Jeff Huntington, Ed Davis, Sharon Luster, Judy Johnson, Desiree Nichol

Special thanks to: Marc Weiss, Nancy Meyer, Jan Rofekamp

Photo Editor: Annie Reichert

Photo credits:
Many of the photographs in this book were generously contributed by the families of *A Lion in the House*. Additional photographs are by Annie Reichert, Melissa Godoy, Susan Zwerdling, Mary Lampson, Julia Reichert, Steven Bognar and other photographers.

Photographs of Steven Bognar and Julia Reichert at the MacDowell Colony © Joanna Eldredge Morrissey

Library of Congress Control Number: 2006925784

Printed in Canada

Table of Contents

Acknowledgements

A Lion in the House was a tremendous team effort on both sides of the camera. Behind the camera and in the cutting room, we found friends and allies who shouldered the responsibility of telling these stories side by side with us. During the years of shooting, there were days when one of us just couldn't be there, or days when we needed an extra camera or someone to record sound. We turned to our colleagues in the small, vital filmmaking community here in Southwest, Ohio, including Barbara Wolf, David Ackels, Thea Lux, Seth Mulliken and Alvoro Leite. They joined us, sometimes on extremely short notice, and under extremely difficult circumstances.

Crucial, too, was the understanding of the people with whom we work at our day jobs. Julia is a film professor at Wright State University. Steve works throughout the state as an artist in the schools. Both of us had colleagues, especially Jim Klein at Wright State and Mary Sheridan at Tussing Elementary School in Pickerington, Ohio, who supported us wholeheartedly when we said, "We need to go to Cincinnati, right now." Or, "I'm at Children's and we just have to keep shooting, so you'll have to take the class alone." They showed no hesitation when they said, "Go."

Though we funded the film ourselves for the first several years, we found early and crucial support from our great home state Ohio Arts Council and from the National Endowment for the Arts.

In the early days of making the film, it found champions though it had yet to find itself. David Davis of Oregon Public Broadcasting, David Liu of the Independent Television Service (ITVS) and Lisa Heller of HBO Documentary gave us confidence and guidance as we worked to keep the film going, and to find funding.

ITVS offered us what every filmmaker can only dream of from a partner—patience. They gave us the time to find the film, and incisive feedback. The ITVS staff are a group of strong individuals who manage to work brilliantly as a unified team. We are especially grateful to Claire Aguilar, Patrick Wickham, Lois Vossen, Klara Grunning-Harris, Jim Sommers, Mary Ann Thyken, Susan Latton, Cindy Burstein, Randall Cole and Dennis Palmieri for their wise shepard-ing of the project.

A turning point in the making of this film came when the Lance Armstrong Foundation got behind the film with its resources and great energy. We'll never forget the breakfast we had in Washington, D.C., with Doug Ulman and Betsy Goldberg, talking about survivorship issues and hearing the news that they were giving the film a major grant.

A few months later, we were back in Washington, thanks to Jay Silver, Pam Jackson and the Intercultural Cancer Council, who invited us to present a clip of the film to an audience of more than 1,000 people at the ICC's Biennial Symposium on Cancer, Minorities and the Medically Underserved. The response to the clip, and the depth of conversation throughout the event, filled us with fire to continue. In the years since, the professionals of the ICC, including Dr. Armin Weinberg and Dr. Lovell Jones, and their compatriots at the National Cancer Institute, including Dr. Emmanuel Taylor, Diana Jeffery, Mary Ann Bright and Dr. Harold Freeman, have continued to educate us about the complexities of health care disparities, and the larger parallels in American society.

We (Julia in particular) have always believed a film is just the beginning. It finds its lasting, concrete value in the way it is used in communities, fosters dialog, organizes stakeholders and builds relationships.

It was through ITVS that a fateful call came, when Jim Sommers contacted us to ask about doing outreach work around *Lion,* to further Julia's goal of seeing the film spark positive social change across the country. None of us could have foreseen how widespread or deep these efforts would run; communities all over the country signed on to work with ITVS and our national partners to offer outreach programs.

As the film began to take shape, we were graced with the dedicated focus and talents of several friends and other students from the Wright State University School of Medicine, young doctors-to-be who shouldered the burden of logging and transcribing the hundreds of hours of tape. Their work, especially that of Dr. Rebecca Podurgiel, Dr. Rama Chandrashekaran and Dr. Kate Conway, helped the telling of this story immensely.

The editing of this film, which in essence is its storytelling, is the result of the work of a small group of filmmakers and editors who day in and day out searched for the truth and heart and poetry within the 525 hours of footage.

The editing process took over five years, and the fellowship of the *Lion*, as we started to call it, saw an evolving membership. Most stayed with the project month after month, reliving deeply emotional, painful situations in the film as they shaped and cut the scenes and sequences. It got harder as we went, but we made it up the mountain side by side with Kevin Jones, Mary Lampson, Jim Klein, Jaime Meyers, Ann Rotolante, Sarah Silver, Brent Huffman, Leilah Weinraub and Beth O'Brien.

We could not have found the film within the footage if not for the honest feedback of friends, colleagues and neighbors who watched rough cuts. Their words helped us see what was not working, where scenes dragged, and so much more. The feedback came from small screenings we did in Yellow Springs and Dayton, Ohio; at ITVS in San Francisco; at the MacDowell Colony in Peterborough, New Hampshire; in Chicago and in Portland, Maine.

Back home, our office and this production have been in the sharp and steady hands of line producer Melissa Godoy, associate producer Karen Durgans, key production assistant Dan Misch and a number of terrific interns from nearby Antioch College.

In the middle years, support both financial and moral came from the Program for Media Artists and the MacDowell Colony. The woods and cabins of MacDowell in particular offered us a safe haven in which to work on some of the hardest parts of the film.

The completion of any film is like the last few miles of a marathon. You're almost there, but every step is ten times harder than when you started. You're exhausted, but the finish line is still up ahead. We only crossed the finish line thanks to the help of our community, to the friends and colleagues who ran along with us, especially John Mays, Amy Cunningham, Eric Johnson, Russ Johnson, Thanos Fatouros, Mike King and the great folks at Glue Edit and Sound One in New York.

As the years passed and the film was in progress, Children's saw changes in both staff and leadership. Yet their support of the film remained, and we are grateful to Dr. Franklin Smith, Director of the Hematology-Oncology Division, to Julia Robertson and to Beth Cullen Canarie, who has been a steady presence since the beginning.

Our colleagues at PBS, and the Corporation for Public Broadcasting understand the potential of *A Lion in the House*, and we're grateful to them, especially Patricia Harrison, Helen Mobley, Jacoba Atlas and Sandy Heberer, for offering and supporting the film's prime-time nationwide broadcast. Locally, we have found great support from Cincinnati's own public television station, CET, and two of its leaders, Susan Howarth and Jack Dominic. Also in Cincinnati, Jay Van Winkle of the Leukemia and Lymphoma Society gave steady support.

Offering tenacious and tireless help in getting the movie out into the world are its distributors Jan Rofekamp and Diana Holtzberg of Films Transit International and wunderkind Jeff Reichert, indie film distributor and beloved nephew of you can guess who.

We are indebted to Margaret McGurk for daring to take on the crafting of this book, for doing such excellent work on such a tight schedule, and for sensitively working with so many participants in *A Lion in the House* to expand and deepen their stories. Luck is when the right person for a challenging job comes along, and we were lucky that Margaret stepped up.

Beyond the aforementioned, and along every step of the way, this project kept going because of the enduring support of friends and colleagues across the country and in our own hometown. There's a thank you list in the end credits of the film. We hope you'll look at it, keeping in mind that each person on that list gave or sacrificed something to help get this film made.

—Steven Bognar & Julia Reichert

My eternal gratitude goes out to Marcy Hawley of Orange Frazer Press for breaking all the rules to see this book into print, and to her colleague Jeff Fulwiler for his wise counsel. Likewise, I am indebted to Dan Misch and Karen Durgans for multiple heroic efforts, and to Lori Stucker for speedy transcription. Jeanette Murray and Rebecca Caires volunteered scrupulous copy editing under taxing circumstances. Any errors herein are mine alone. For priceless moral support and encouragement, I thank Charles Mueller and my personal board of female advisors. This book would not have been created unless Steven Bognar, Julia Reichert and Melissa Godoy decided to ignore impossible odds and commit themselves to making it happen. Above all, it owes its existence to the courage and generosity of the families who opened their hearts for *A Lion in the House*.

—*Margaret A. McGurk*

***A Lion in the House* was created with major support from:**

itvs
independent television service

CDC
SAFER • HEALTHIER • PEOPLE

LANCE ARMSTRONG
FOUNDATION

NATIONAL
ENDOWMENT
FOR THE ARTS

Ohio Arts Council
A STATE AGENCY
THAT SUPPORTS PUBLIC
PROGRAMS IN THE ARTS

The **Program** for **Media Artists**

The **MacDowell** Colony

A Lion in the House is a co-production with the Independent Television Service, Executive Producer Sally Jo Fifer. Funding from the Corporation for Public Broadcasting.

Foreword

Imagine going through one of the hardest things you could ever face, struggling to save the life of your child. Now imagine being asked to go through this on camera.

Imagine yourself a nurse or doctor struggling to save the lives of kids, often facing great uncertainty, yet charged with showing leadership, compassion and confidence. The choices you recommend, the words you use, have life and death consequences. Now imagine being asked to do this job on camera.

Imagine yourself in the leadership of an award-winning hospital, and you're being asked by one of your divisions to give a film crew almost unlimited access to make an independent documentary that the hospital won't control.

Well, this happened. It began at the end of the last century, in Cincinnati, Ohio, a Midwestern city on a curve of the Ohio River, when Dr. Robert Arceci, then director of the Hematology/Oncology Division at Cincinnati Children's Hospital Medical Center proposed that a documentary be made about what a family experiences when a child is fighting cancer.

Almost nine years later, the documentary *A Lion in the House* emerged into the world. Much work went into its filming and editing. Much support came from the world of public television, from the cancer support community and from the community we call home. Many outreach projects and efforts have grown from the film. But none of this would have happened if three parties, three groups of individuals, had not taken a profound leap of faith.

Two of the groups are professionals—the folks who run Cincinnati Children's Hospital Medical Center, and the caregivers who work in the Hematology-Oncology Division. The administrators took a leap of faith in giving access to their hospital to two independent filmmakers they did not know or control. In essence, they were putting the image and reputation of the hospital at risk. It's a testament to their confidence in the excellence of their institution that they opened their doors to us.

The same is true on an individual level for every nurse, every doctor, every aide, social worker, psychologist, nutritionist, school intervention expert, child life specialist and for every other professional working with the families who fight cancer at Cincinnati Children's.

It's too easy to think of these folks as a faceless class of professionals doing their jobs. They are also moms and dads, husbands, wives, friends and neighbors who come to work to take care of kids who might die.

They are nurses like Linda, Connie, Melinda, Sally, Rebecca, Nikki, Kim, Sherri, Sandy, David, Dan and Mark, or doctors like Cyndi, Claire, Paul, Ted, Fred, Vinod, Karen, Joe, Ralph, Bob, and many more who work the long shifts, day and night, on the fourth of July, on Thanksgiving Day and Christmas Eve.

Each one pours heart and head, soul and spirit into this work. They get close to these kids. They get close to these parents. And every year, they lose children they have struggled to save. Each one took the leap of faith to be part of these stories.

The greatest leap of faith was made by the parents of the kids at the heart of *Lion*. They took a leap by letting us film, month after month, year after year, especially when things began to go badly for some of the kids. They made the specific choice to say, "Yes, I will share this with the world, though it may be the hardest thing I ever go through." It's hard to overstate the generosity of such a decision.

Now, years later, that generosity feels even greater than we imagined. When *A Lion in the House* premiered at the 2006 Sundance Film Festival (where it was honored to be the longest film ever chosen for the documentary competition), audiences met members from all five families in the film, and with five of their key caregivers.

What none of us anticipated, save perhaps the parents who lost their children, was the overwhelming challenge of watching the film again in a public setting. For these parents, seeing their children first charm, then steal the hearts of hundreds of people had its own bittersweet power. As each child's onscreen journey grew harder, the mom, dad, sister or brother of that child—knowing the storms to come—watched the audience hold on to hope. To relive those hardships was profoundly difficult. To then step in front of the audience and engage in discussion was heroic.

A Lion in the House was not easy to make, but we've received such tremendous support and gratitude that we want to send that support, that gratitude back where it belongs.

To Dr. Robet J. Arceci, whose vision and commitment led to this film becoming real, thank you.

To the individuals at Cincinnati Children's who gave us access, who entrusted us with the great name of their institution, thank you.

To the doctors and nurses who taught us the ropes, who gave us advice, who set up a cot for us to catch a few hours sleep, who tolerated our camera and our questions year in and year out, thank you.

But above all, to the families—to Justin, Jennifer, Adam, Debbie, Susan, Shelly, Dale, Tim, Taletha, Tyrik, Marietha, Ron, Alex, Jackie, Brittany, Judy, Scott, Alex, Regina, Jennifer, Natalie, Beth, Frank, the grammas, grandpas, uncles, aunts and cousins—who trusted us with their stories, year after year, who trusted us with their challenges, their uncertainty, their turmoil, their hearts and the most precious thing of all, their children, thank you.

—Steven Bognar and Julia Reichert

Introduction

"Childhood cancer occurs regularly, randomly and spares no social, economic or ethnic groups."
—*Hope Street Kids*

"You know you are truly alive when you are living among lions."
—*Isak Dinesen.*

Steven Bognar and Julia Reichert did not know in early 1997 when they were invited to shoot a documentary about cancer patients at Cincinnati Children's Hospital Medical Center that they were about to make a war movie.

Yet that is exactly what emerged over the next six years as they followed Tim Woods, Alexandra Lougheed, Justin Ashcraft, Jennifer Moone, Alex Fields and their families into battle against a ferocious enemy.

Any thinking human understands that having a child with cancer hurts. *A Lion in the House* shows how it hurts.

Cancer kills without reason or mercy. It spreads the incurable virus of grief. It scars survivors and those who love them. A uniquely aggressive enemy, it can lurk undetected for years. Apparently vanquished, it may only be in temporary retreat. Battle lines shift endlessly. One advance is met with a relapse; new weapons can cause side effects as fearsome as any malignancy.

Yet, the disease also inspires bravery, generosity, compassion and family bonds that no ordinary life can match. It taps unsuspected reserves of hope, resilience, determination, even humor, in children and parents. It drives scientists to test the limits of their skill in the search for a cure. As Dr. Arceci told the filmmakers, "I see very little burnout amongst pediatric oncologists. Because kids are dying, I see people staying in the profession, not leaving it."

The American Cancer Society estimated that in 2006 some 9,500 children up to age 14 would be diagnosed with cancer and 1,560 would die. In 1997, when filming on *A Lion in the House* was getting under way, the number of new cases was about 8,800, but the number of deaths 1,700.

What those statistics show is that lives are being saved in greater numbers, year by year, as scientists create an ever-growing stockpile of weapons to fight malignancies. The ACS reports that, overall, the death rate among children with cancer is almost half of what it was in 1975.

Physicians and scientists shy away from the word "cure," given the risk that apparently quashed cancers can reappear years later. Instead, they count the number of patients who are still alive five years after diagnosis as the benchmark for long-term survival. Before 1970, only 50 percent of juvenile cancer patients in the U.S. lived that long; today, the survival rate is 80 percent.

Dr. Robert Arceci, then head of pediatric oncology at Cincinnati Children's, understood those numbers as well as anyone in the country when he contacted Steve and Julia to present his idea of recording the unvarnished truth about childhood cancer, a dream he had harbored for years.

He did not know the irony of his request. Shortly before his call, Julia's daughter, Lela, had completed her last treatment for Hodgkin's Lymphoma. Julia and Steve, who have shared a home as well as a professional partnership for more than 15 years, reacted from the gut: We don't want to do this. It took only brief reflection for them to change their minds. They knew instinctively how important the project could be.

July 4, 1997, was the first day of shooting, when they brought their camera to the backyard of the Lougheed family home to capture Alexandra and her sister Jackie frolicking in the back yard. As the months unfolded and they met the children, their families, their doctors and nurses, the filmmakers became, in essence, members of an extended clan dedicated to supporting young patients.

Steve and Julia had no idea how intensely the project would affect them. They did not know it would consume their lives for eight years of filming and editing.

They witnessed the toll that chemotherapy and radiation take on the body. They stood by as families faced impossible choices between harrowing treatments or allowing cancer to take its inexorable toll. They saw some of their young friends succumb to the lethal side effects of the powerful anti-cancer drug Methotrexate.

Steve and Julia recorded the conflicts, the confusion, the anger surrounding extreme decisions. They saw how the catastrophic disease can break hearts and undermine religious faith, marriages, family ties, finances and careers.

They also saw the enormous spirit of the children and the boundless love of their families. Over and over, they saw parents, siblings and patients stand up to the ordeal of treatment and emerge undiminished. Perhaps the most vivid image of their collective triumphs was the day when Beth Moone, who had seen her little girl through successful treatment for leukemia, celebrated her survival by running the Chicago Marathon.

In addition to personal experiences, *A Lion in the House* opens a window on some of the larger social issues surrounding life-threatening childhood illness.

Despite enormous efforts to ensure that every child can get the best care, money still matters. Less money means fewer options and bigger bureaucratic burdens.

Survivors also may find they are unprepared for years of physical and emotional fallout. As the number of children cured of cancer rises, evidence is mounting that unexpected health issues arise when survivors reach adulthood.

Yet despite its fearsome cost, the war on cancer is fueled by hope. Every day, research opens doors that can lead to new treatments, even cures, despite sharp reductions in public funding. Scores of private organizations pour enormous energy into raising money to supplement research, and to provide education, services and comfort. Medical professionals devote their lives to winning daily battles to advance the science of pediatric oncology, with boundless compassion for the human beings in their care.

Behind all of these efforts is an army of children who will not be defined, nor defeated, by a fearsome disease.

This book contains a series of first-person accounts from families and some of the medical professionals who helped them. In narratives compiled from interviews during and after filming, they talk about what they learned from the experiences captured in the movie.

The pediatric cancer unit at Cincinnati Children's—one of the world's largest pediatric hospitals—was known as 5A during filming. It is where much of the movie takes place, and where the young patients and their families learned to take part in their own care, in preparation for the day they can go home. They learned how to keep medical supplies sterile, how to change dressings, how to look after what are called C-lines—surgically implanted central catheters for delivering intravenous chemotherapy and taking blood samples. Parents, said one of the doctors, "end up with skills a nurse would envy."

Families also learned to deal with a large and changing cast of medical caregivers. On any given day, they could see an attending physician (who directs the case), one or more fellows (physicians involved in advanced specialty training and research), a few residents (physicians in the final stage of clinical training), and a handful of medical students. As is common in teaching hospitals, the attendings doctors, fellows and residents regularly rotate to different parts of the hospital—a situation the families often found confusing.

Only the nurses stay in the unit, and spent the most time looking after patients day-to-day. Not surprisingly, they often developed the closest emotional bonds with the children and became the families' most trusted source for information.

Alongside the family recollections in this book, Steve, Julia, and their colleagues talk about how they made the documentary, as well as their relationships with the movie's subjects.

Many people who appear in *A Lion in the House* were on hand when it debuted at the 2006 Sundance Film Festival in Park City, Utah. Patients, parents, siblings and doctors joined the filmmakers to see, for the first time, how audiences responded to their stories. What they saw stunned them. Tears, laughter, standing ovations and the affection of viewers who saw themselves in the struggles on screen.

The response of Sundance audiences assured the survivors that they had done the right thing to open their lives and hearts to the cameras, and reminded them that they are not alone. This book is intended to do the same, for everyone who has suffered through childhood cancer, for friends and families of the stricken, for medical professionals who care for them.

Most of all, it speaks to everyone who learns from Tim, Alexandra, Justin, Jennifer and Alex what it is to live with a lion in the house.

Chapter 1

Justin ASHCRAFT

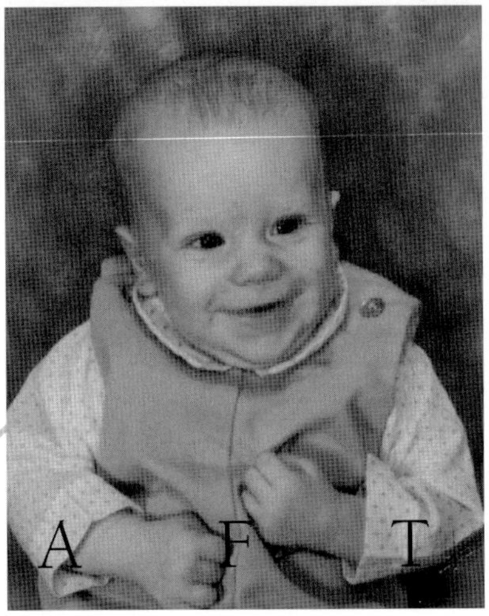

Justin Ashcraft is the youngest of three children. His mom, Debbie, says he was ornery from the start.

debbieKENNER

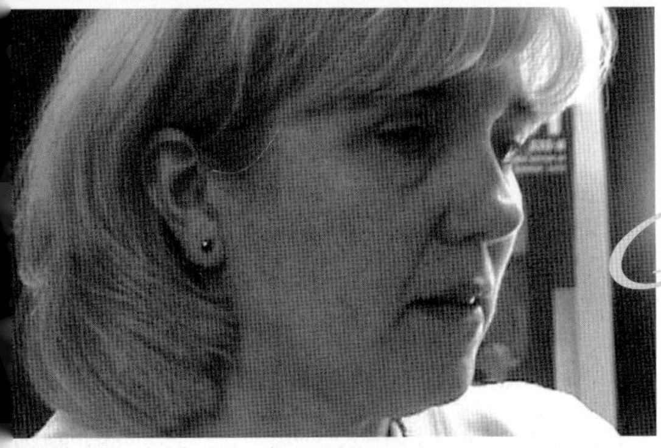

Debbie, Justin's mom, devoted her life to her son's care for over nine years. She was like a mother lion.

Justin's mother, Debbie Kenner, was married to his father, Dale Ashcraft, at the time the youngest of their three children was diagnosed. She and Dale later divorced and both remarried. She still lives in Northern Kentucky.

The day before he was diagnosed he was home with something like the flu. The next day he got up and I sent him on to school. I went to work. Justin's father was at work. The school nurse called and said that Justin wasn't feeling well. An hour went by and she called again. He was having severe leg cramps. I thought, "Is it the flu thing going on from the day before? Or, his brother was tall, is he getting growing pains?" I made an appointment for the pediatrician immediately after work. The pediatrician sent us on to St. Elizabeth just for blood work. I didn't know this at the time, but he thought that he might have diabetes. The doctor said that I could go back to work. He said, "When I find out the lab results, I'll call you."

My husband called me at work and said the doctor wanted both of us back at his office. I could tell, of course, that it was bad news. He said, "From this point on, I will no longer be your pediatrician." This was the pediatrician that I had since my oldest was two. He said, "You need to go immediately to Children's Hospital." I can't remember him saying anything about leukemia. That part did not even register to me. I remember he said, "Don't go home, don't get clothes, don't do anything but get there immediately." So that's what we did. Justin's white count at that time was 180,000. (Normal white cell count is between 4,000 and 11,000 per cubic millimeter of blood.)

Everything went so fast. That night they transfused him. My girlfriend was a nurse and she stayed with me. She told me exactly what was going to go on, 'cause that is fearful—being in ICU and watching the blood being pulled out of him and put back in. He had a severe reaction to the blood product. They had to put him on Benadryl and I don't know what else. He was nothing but hives. He was a mess. He was solid red.

My husband was out there and we would take shifts in the waiting room. It was quite an ordeal that night. If we had not gotten him there, he would have died the next day. We learned that later.

I am sure that day someone sat down with us and told us it was leukemia. I cannot recollect that at all. I remember sitting down with a hematologist and him going through different treatment protocols that Children's had to offer. We had to decide what we wanted him to go on. That is a lot. I know the hematologist sat down with us for like two hours. We were in total shock.

I wish now if I had anything to do over, I wish that we would have gone with a stronger regimen. I feel that with leukemia in boys, you have got to hit it with all you have got and hope to God they can make it through.

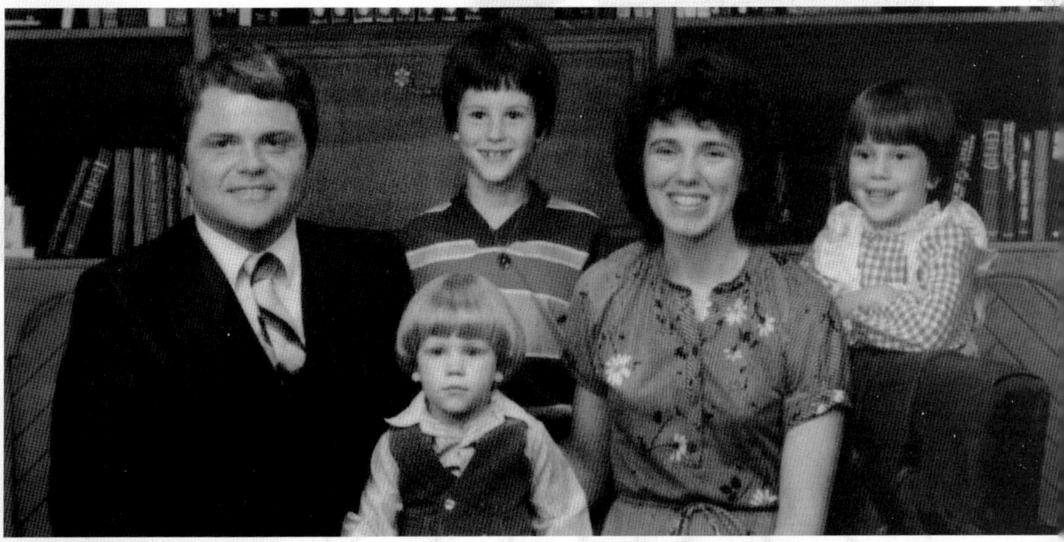

The Ashcrafts in 1982 could have no inkling of what was to befall their family.

He went through a lot, but he was very fortunate that he was not in a hospital a lot for different things to do with chemo. He lived a pretty normal life even though he was going through the chemotherapy.

Justin would have chemo, come home, cut the grass, ride his bike. He would be sick all the way home, vomiting in the car. As a child, I had been very sickly. I swore that when I grew up and had children that I would not dote and smother them about a medical problem. It killed me to see him go out and cut the grass, to hardly be able to push the lawnmower, but that is what he wanted to do. It's not that I made him do it.

Whenever he would get chemo, on the way to the hospital we never discussed what treatment he was going to get. He knew the night before. We would talk about it. "Do I have to get a spinal tap tomorrow?" "Yes, you do." That would be the end of the con-

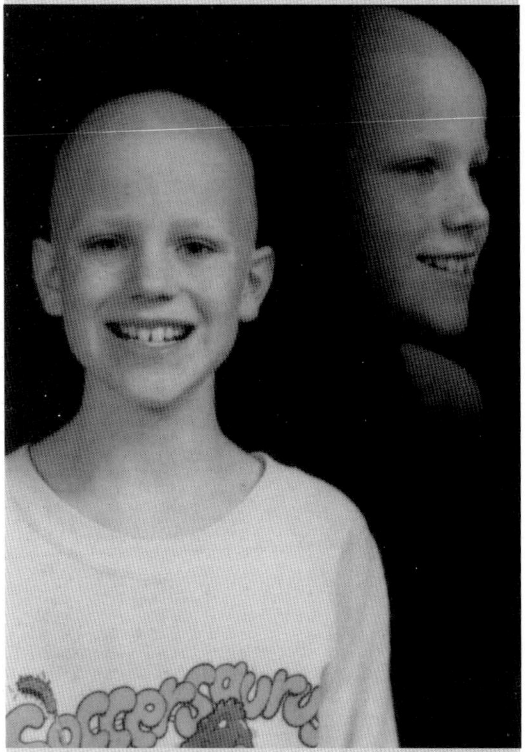

Justin's 4th grade class picture.

versation. He would be real quiet going to the hospital. If he wanted to talk I figured he would say something to me.

He knew what had to be done. I didn't cry over him. I didn't say, "Oh, poor Justin's getting a shot. This is going to hurt you." Be positive. Don't go dwelling over needles. That is the worst thing you can ever do to a child. Yeah, they have to get the shot. They know they have to get the shot. Once they get the shot it is going to be fine. That is the way we were from day one when he was nine years old.

This is the way I was from day one with this illness: Be positive. Don't dwell on things. Go forward. Never look back. That is the way we always were. I think that is why he lived as long as he did. I never said, "Lord, why me?" I never blamed Him.

We would go to Virginia to the National Cancer Institute. When you got a spinal tap, you got put out totally. Justin was like, "I'm not getting put out for a stupid spinal tap." He didn't even take the cream they put on your back to numb it. He was like, "I don't know what you are talking about. I never got that stuff where I'm from. You take it like a man!" They were horrified. They called him the bionic kid.

Justin hated to be put asleep. He liked to be conscious and wanted to know what was going on with him. He wanted you to be upfront with him. "Let's not beat around the bush. I want to know." That is just the way we always handled it.

He was ornery the day the kid was born. When he was two, he fell and had to get stitches. On the way home, he pulled the stitches out. I lost him in McAlpin's Department Store. He would get under the rack. I'd have a terrible time trying to find him. Scared the heck out of me. He was just an ornery child. He was still, growing up. The kids, my other two, would feud continuously. Like brothers and sisters. Justin would get the attention, of course. They would tease him, tease him tremendously. Of course, that used to drive me absolutely crazy.

I would tell parents that when there are other children, include them. We did not include them. I didn't realize it. Adam was fifteen, Jennifer was twelve. We figured with them being as old as they were, they could handle being left alone a lot because I was at the hospital all the time.

At one point, Justin got tickets for Disney. There were four tickets. Adam got excluded because he went to Disney with his

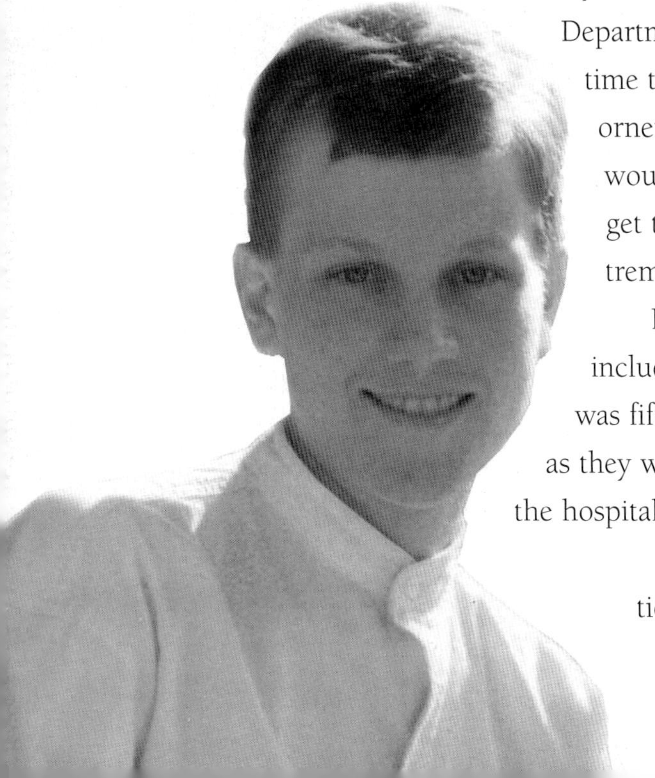

Justin was proud to graduate high school, though over the years he missed a lot of days and had few good friends at school.

friends a few months before. We figured, okay, we couldn't afford to take him. We just didn't have the money. But the family was not together, the whole family. I never realized that hurt him. You just don't, you have so much going on.

Justin was the youngest. With him to come down with an illness and the other kids are a little older, I just assumed that they could take all that. Don't assume. It affected Adam so much. I never realized it, not until just a couple of years ago when the kids and I sat down. Jennifer would say how much it bothered her to stay with this person and that person. Bring your kids in on it too. They are a part of it. Do not exclude them. I really regret that. It bothers me.

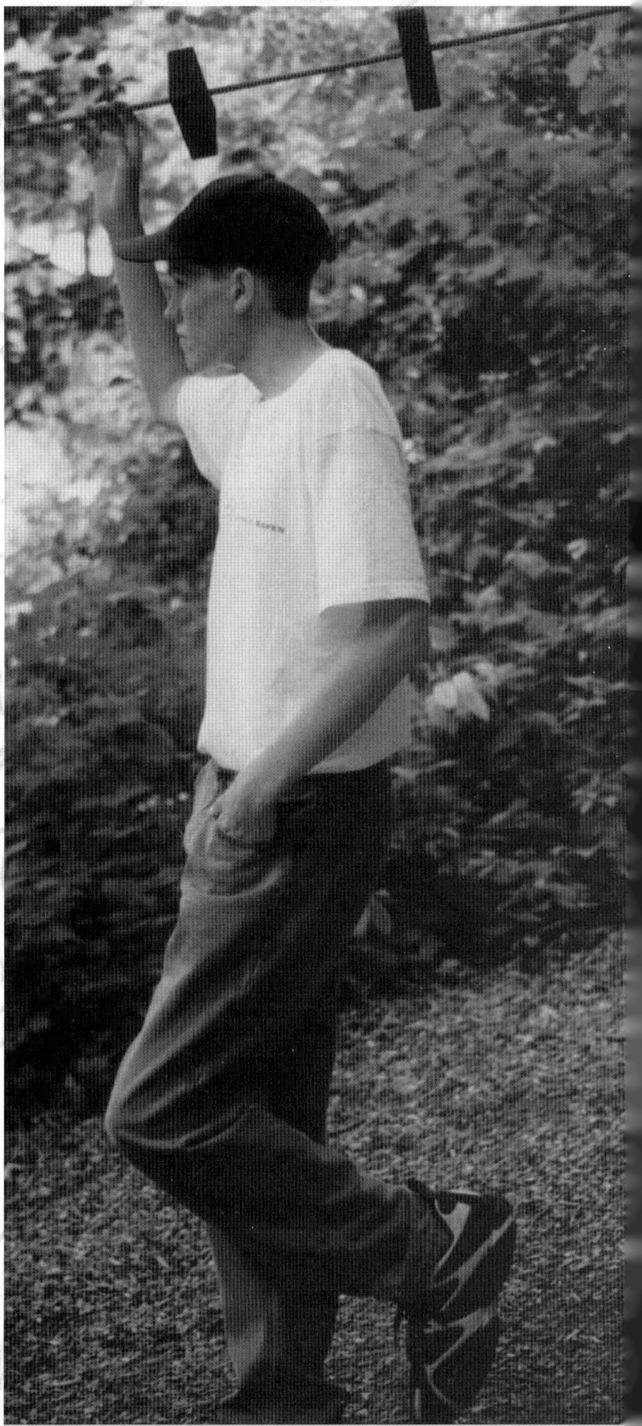

Justin loved going to cancer camp. For most kids, camp is a time to feel like a normal kid. But a rare spider bite at camp almost led Justin to disaster.

Justin never wanted school kids to know anything about his problem. He hated the fact that they brought it up. Children's Hospital always wanted the schoolchildren to know what was going on with him.

The sad part about Justin growing up in the age that he was, he never had kids his own age to hang with. He never went to the prom. We were in a Children's study group on how classmates would react to kids with cancer. Justin said he was treated real nice, but he was never included in anything. He always felt like he was different.

He would feel more normal when he would go to cancer camp. We always called it cancer camp. He always went to Camp Friendship in Lebanon until he became a teenager. The year before he died, his thing was to be a counselor. He wanted to be a counselor really bad. Of course, he never got that far.

I was scared to death the first year that I sent him. I knew there would be nurses from Children's there. If you needed chemo or anything, they were there. Here you have a kid with cancer sick on chemo, spiking fevers, and you are sending him off to camp. You have to open up windows with no screens. They are having a fly-killing contest. Germs! You are thinking they are going in such a germ-thriving environment. He loved every minute of it. If they got real scared, they could call. Mom is sitting by the phone. He never called. He was gone for three days. It killed me that first year. He'd come home and ramble on and on and on. He couldn't wait to go back the next year.

To me, children that have cancer are so beyond their age group. They've had to grow up real quick. Life to them—they

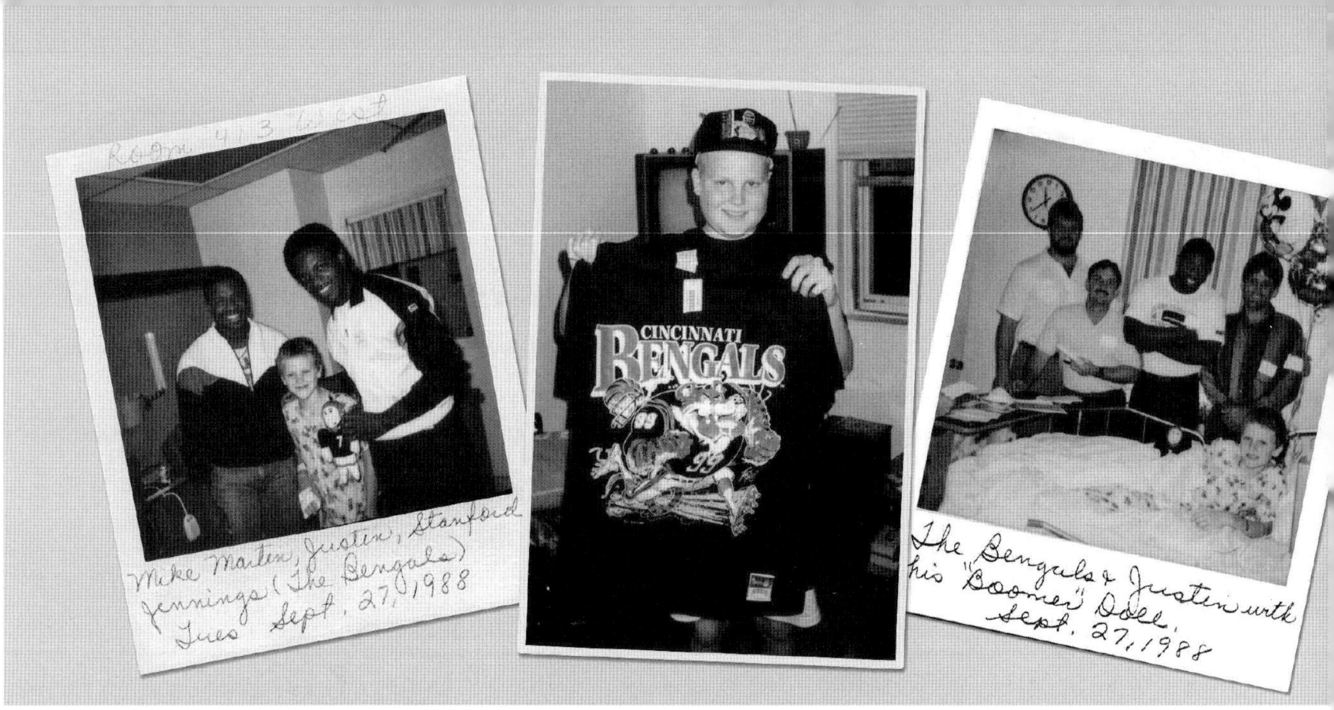

The Bengals and the Reds adopted Justin. He became a "poster child" for leukemia. He loved the attention!

don't take life for granted like teenagers do. It's very important to them. They want to live it.

Justin was a special child. He knew so many people. He knew Cindy Crawford. He went out to Colorado twice and was involved in the Silver Lining Ranch. That is where he met Cindy Crawford. (Tennis star) Andrea Yeager was also a close friend of his. While he was dying, Andrea called to talk to him. His head turned towards the phone. Those are the things I will never ever forget.

Bob Huggins (University of Cincinnati basketball coach) was just fantastic with my son. He got to go into practices. Now if they lost a game, he was banned from the locker room because of all the yelling and screaming.

The president of the Leukemia & Lymphoma Society at the time, Max Wiseman, he had a brother who died of leukemia. He was around my age, and Cathy Sprankel who ran to raise funds for the Leukemia Society, those two were Justin's best friends. They would take him to the Reds' game and to the UC games. Marty (Brenneman) and Joe (Nuxhall) were very close friends of Justin's. We had Marty's phone number at home if we wanted to call.

(Former Bengals coach) Sam Wyche was a wonderful friend. (Former Reds star) Chris Sabo, we have pictures with him. When Justin was first diagnosed that first week, Stanley Jennings came from the Bengals with Mike Martin; both guys cried in Justin's room. I'll never forget that. It really touched them. They really cried.

I just can't say enough. News plays out the bad side of people, but when there is a devastating illness like my son's, I had so many good people helping us.

We heard about the film when Dr. Arceci came to us and mainly asked Justin, I guess because of his age, if he would like to participate in a film that would help children in his situation and help families cope with it. He never said no. I never did either. He was all for it. He was a big ham.

Boy, Steve and Julia were "up our butt" always. But no, the cameras never bothered me because I was helping someone else. I hoped to God that they could look and benefit from whatever we were doing.

Justin was dying and someone brought us in all kinds of goodies in the room. I was alone on New Year's Eve. That was when he had his brain surgery. Everyone left. The film crew came back and stayed with me past midnight. I will never forget that as long as I live. Not to feel sorry for yourself, but that was not the time to be alone.

I cannot wait for the premiere to see other people's reaction and hope to God that it will do good. I cannot say enough about Julia and Steve. Steve and Justin started a relationship right from day one. I don't know if it is because Justin was so into movies. They just clicked. Steve and Julia, they're a great couple. I cannot say enough about them.

I cannot wait to see Alex (Lougheed's) family. Alex's dad reminds me so much of me. Coming away from the film, Alex bothered me more than anything because of the fact that was a family that touched me from day one. She was around the corner from Justin.

I know it was at least seven times that he relapsed. He went through a bone marrow transplant where my daughter was the donor. He was fine for eighteen months with no leukemia cells. A cure isn't the answer. The quality of life is. Will you ever be cancer free? There are so many people, they have breast cancer and they are "cured," but three years later they have another cancer somewhere else. I don't know. If I had it all to do over, I would not strive for that ultimate cure. I would just strive to keep him alive.

His leukemia was rare. What was told to us at the time was that one out of 600 leukemia kids ever got it in their spinal fluid. His was not in his blood. It was in the beginning, but then he had radiation. Somehow, because of that it ended up being in the spinal fluid. This is what his doctor believes. It is hard to pinpoint who's right and who's wrong. I never did really kind of blame anybody for that part. When they found it in his spinal fluid, he got an Omia reservoir. It was a rubbery egg-shaped thing inserted in his head. That is where he got his chemo injected.

We ended up going to Houston (for a clinical trial). I stayed there for a month for him to get this new chemo drug that he was going to get through St. Jude. St. Jude refused to give him the drug because he did not meet their criteria. They could not find cancer cells in his fluid.

(Justin relapsed again in late 1998. His primary doctor, who was about to leave the city for a new job, recommended a powerful combination of three chemotherapy drugs in an effort to control his leukemia. The drugs probably caused lesions in his brain and paralysis.)

At the very end when we exhausted everything, we went back to the first injection that he had that more or less did him in. There were three drugs in one injection. After the first injection, he was stumbling. I had to make the decision whether to go on after that. If we did go on, we didn't know what would happen. He was all for it.

Claire Mazewski, his main doctor, left towards the end when we were on experimental drugs. When you are going through an experimental drug with the National Cancer Institute, you go by the book. He was taken off of that drug

Justin's Grandma Rita shared the house with Debbie and Justin. She was fierce in her protection of Justin.

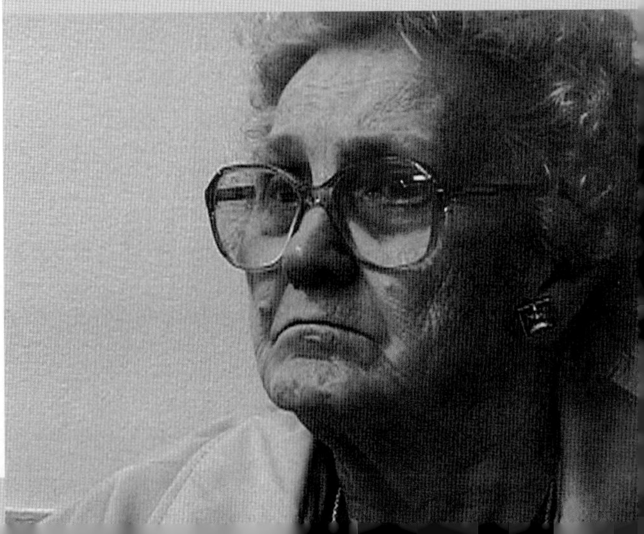

because they said that he had four leukemia cells and was no longer a candidate. His doctor was gone. I fought with them on that. He could have stayed on that protocol, but Claire was not there to fight for me. Somebody else was there. From that day on it was not good.

I should have asked her, "Being a mother, would you go on with the second injection?" That was how close we were; I knew she had children. I wish now I would have just stopped and not done the second injection. That totally paralyzed him.

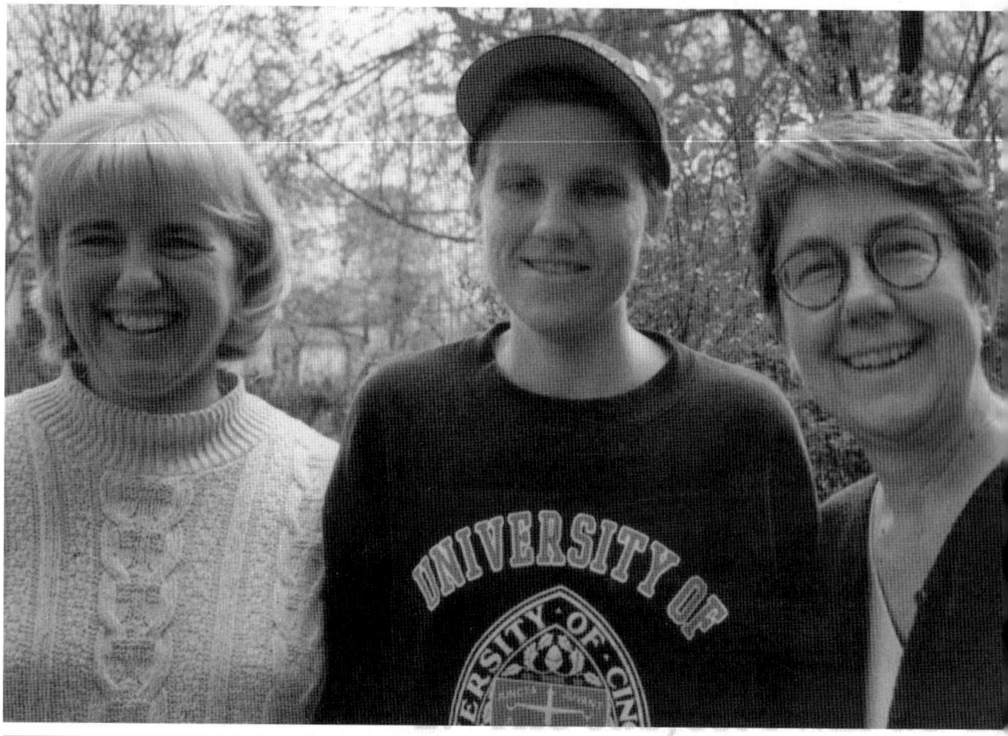

Justin and Debbie visited Julia and Steven in their little town of Yellow Springs. This was the last day the filmmakers ever saw Justin walk.

He was taken from his room to the ICU and put on a bypass machine. You'll see in the film where I'm going there (the morning Justin went to the ICU). I am just disoriented. I always tried to be in total control of what was going on with him.

I hated him being on a machine. I promised him that he would never be put onto a breathing machine. I fought with ICU. At the moment, I thought my child was dying, and yes, he was. The more and more that he became alert and on that machine, it kept coming back to me that this was not what I promised. They kept saying, "You know, he'll die if he's not on this." I said, "Well, let it be."

I don't remember how many days he was in ICU. He was not there long on that machine. I said, "Whatever will be, will be, but if he's going to die, he'll be dying downstairs on 5A, the floor where it all began. "I wanted him around the nurses that took care of him. I wanted all the support that I could get from the nurses. That was our family." They kept saying, "As soon as you get him in the elevator (from ICU to 5A), he will die." They prepared for that. He lived a month and a half after they said that. They don't know everything.

When we were in ICU (when Justin was first diagnosed), I got really close (to another family). I don't even know the child's name; the father was always by his side. We got to become really good friends just through that. He knew his son was not going to live, so he gave us his son's teddy bear. I still have his white teddy bear. People just really touch you.

My biggest fear with Justin with leukemia was a little girl that was across from us. She bled from every hole imaginable in her body for days. The family would not give up hope and kept okaying her to get blood. As fast as they were putting the blood in, it was coming out. I can remember that to this day. The nurses were coming out crying about how she was bleeding profusely. I did not want to see my child like that. I could not have stood it. That is what I remember when I think of leukemia and dying with it.

The way Justin died, I wasn't there, but he was peaceful. Even the month and a half that he lasted, he was peaceful. I read to him every night. He loved Mark Maguire and Sammy Sosa. The book I read, you read it one way and read about Mark Maguire. Then you flipped the book and could read about Sammy Sosa. I always heard that even when you are in a comatose state that they can still hear you.

The youth people at the hospital gave me a boom box to use. Dave Matthews was his favorite singer, so I played Dave Matthews. Every time Dave played, you could see the oxygen levels on his monitor going up. I played it the day before he died.

Even being twenty, he never shaved a day in his life. He always had a little peach fuzz. Well, wearing an oxygen mask for a couple of months, you grow hair. You grow a lot of hair. Dr. Arceci came in the day before he died. He brought in a little can of shaving cream. He said, "Will you please do me one favor and shave that child? He is a man and he needs to be shaved."

By God, we shaved him. With the nurses, we cranked up the music and his numbers were going through the roof. We had the best time. I know and hope that Justin inside had the best time. I know this sounds morbid, but the day he died at least he was clean-shaven.

I firmly believe that Justin fed off of Dale's and my energy totally. I had no doubts about that whatsoever. We never gave up on him and he fed off of that. I would have liked to have been there for that moment. Did it bother me that I wasn't? No, that was Justin. That is just the way he would have wanted it.

It was hard, but my faith got stronger than ever. I was brought up Catholic and married into Union Presbyterian Church. That is where I went with Justin all through this. They were fantastic. Now that I am remarried, my husband is Baptist, which is neither here nor there. As long as you believe in the Lord, that is all that counts.

We weren't every week church-going people. My faith was very, very strong. When I was in grade school you went to church every day before school. That was just the way it was. One year my cousin gave Justin a teenage Bible. She gave it to him for his birthday and nothing else was brought up. Well, I went down to his room one day, and sitting there wide open was the Bible. I was just ecstatic.

(At one point, a friend invited Debbie and Justin to a service with a minister known as a faith healer. Late in the service, Justin approached the minister and Debbie followed him.)

The minister is already over by Justin. He asked Justin why he was there. Justin said, "I have leukemia. Everything has failed that we have been trying to do. I'm going to St. Jude's in a couple weeks for a cure." He said, "Son, I'll tell you one thing. Whatever I do in front of you I am not going to harm you in any way. Do you believe in God?" Justin said, "Yes, I do."

The minister said a prayer. With his hand, I thought he shoved him because of the way it looked. He was in front of me and I didn't know what was going on. Justin collapsed, hit the floor. Church people were all around him. I'm looking down at Justin, and he is just smiling and beaming. He said, "Mom, I'm fine."

The minister looked at me and smiled, "You must be his mom." Again he said, "Do you mind if I say a prayer? I know you need what I am going to give you." He prayed and he blew on me. I hit the floor. I hit the floor with such force. Again church people were there. They prayed over us and immediately we just got back up. The service seemed like in two seconds it was over. This is going into eleven thirty at night. We went on home. Justin and I rode together in the car. It was like, well I know the Holy Spirit was with us. We were beaming. We were laughing. I felt like I was totally drunk. We laughed like people just kept telling us jokes. It was dark out, but to us it could have been the brightest, most beautiful day, like we were on the ocean. That is just the way we felt.

Other families, when their children are deceased, they say they have appeared or had a feeling. When Justin died I couldn't wait for the feeling. I'm like, okay it's time. I'd go past his room to go do the laundry. His boombox, I would play his music. His CDs are still in there. I've never changed his music. I'd be down there and hoping for him to present himself just one more time. Not a thing, nothing.

Then one day I was down in the basement doing the laundry and I felt funny. I wasn't thinking about Justin. It had been several years since he passed. As I turned to the right, by God, he was leaning up against the cabinet with his arm to his head laughing at me, biggest smile on his face and shaking his head. He was always like, "Oh, God, Mom what are you coming up with next?" That is exactly the way he was.

I was kind of in shock. I didn't know how to react. I wanted to hold the moment. I did a double take and then he was gone. It was that quick and that was all. What a wonderful feeling, and for him to be smiling. I just hold the moment and hang on to it.

(Debbie and Dale now have three grandchildren, Sidney, Cameron, and Ian)

I absolutely love to be a grandma. It's the most wonderful feeling in the world. And Cameron is so cute. She has come out of her shell. When she sees me now it's "Grandma!" She has to sit by me.

I love my grandchild to death but I don't want to be with my grandchild every day.

I want to get beyond my family; I feel like my family's okay now. We were really united as one for so long. I never gave it a thought about what I was going to do tomorrow. It's hard, it's really hard to think, at my age, what's going to happen.

Whatever happens, I hope it takes place that I do make a difference in this world. I keep hearing Justin in the background. I feel like he made a difference to so many lives and I want a part of me to do the same. I don't know how that's going to turn out. I don't know how I'm going to make that happen, but I don't want to be just another human being. I want to make a difference.

daleASHCRAFT

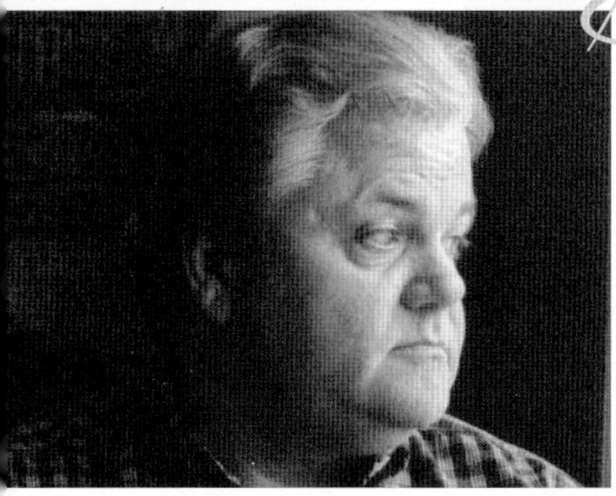

Dale Ashcraft two years after Justin's death.

Dale Ashcraft and his wife Susan Ashcraft still live in Northern Kentucky.

I was working and they called me to tell me he had called. I picked him up and took him home, and we went to the doctor. We went to see his doctor (who said), "I think we need to get some tests done." He was always known as a doctor who would do tests beyond what he should. The nurses used to make fun of him. We went and got the blood work done. We went home. Then, he called and said, "Mr. Ashcraft, it's leukemia. You need to go to Childrens."

I would have rather gone totally stupid into it. I wouldn't want to have known what these kids go through.

People that have gone through it helped a lot. This was before the Internet took off too. It was kind of an unexact science. Everybody had different kinds of cancer. You'd try to get as much knowledge as quickly as you could get it. Doctors would set you down and go over this, this, and this, but they were really busy and had a lot going on with a lot of kids. With the parents, you got the inside view of what to expect.

You didn't know what experiments were going on. You didn't know there was another experiment in Albuquerque or an experiment at the Mayo. Things were not communicated. Now you can go out there and know almost every clinical trial out there in the world. You can go out there and investigate. In those days, you were really on your own. I think they have come a long way.

You learn more how to deal with children and their problems. With the leukemia situation, it really amazed me about how strong kids are. I always said that about Justin, too. It changes you. We went through hell, boy. A piece of you dies.

After Debbie and I got divorced in '92 *(Justin lived with his mother and grandma)*, our big deal—his and mine—was that we'd go to the movies at least once a week or we'd go for miniature golf or something like that. Justin never had much of a social life because he was always sick. He didn't have much of the social skills like a lot of other kids his age.

I took my three kids on a cruise. I took Jennifer the first year, then I took Adam and Justin the second year. It was only a four-day cruise to the Bahamas, to a private island. Adam had social skills, so after the first day I didn't see him for most of the cruise. I'd see him at dinner at night. For Justin, they had a thing for teenage kids, so I suggested that we go down and look. I said, "Here it is. Go on." Justin asked, "Do I have to?" "Yes." He went in for a second and came back to say, "I'll see you later." There were two teenage girls in there and another teenage boy.

What's funny is one time I went in to see him at Children's and he was going through some really big-time problems. I forget what he had. That kid had so many IVs, I'm surprised he had any arms left after all those years. He was a tiny kid, in a ton of pain. Every parent says it to his or her kid, "I wish I could do it for you." He looked over and said, "You couldn't take it."

Even as good as a lot of the care was, Justin was very good about watching the meds that they gave him. If they sent someone in to give a bone marrow aspiration, he would do that without anesthetic. If they were in the middle of it and they screwed it up, he would stop them right in the middle and have them get someone that knew what they were doing. It was kind of the way you

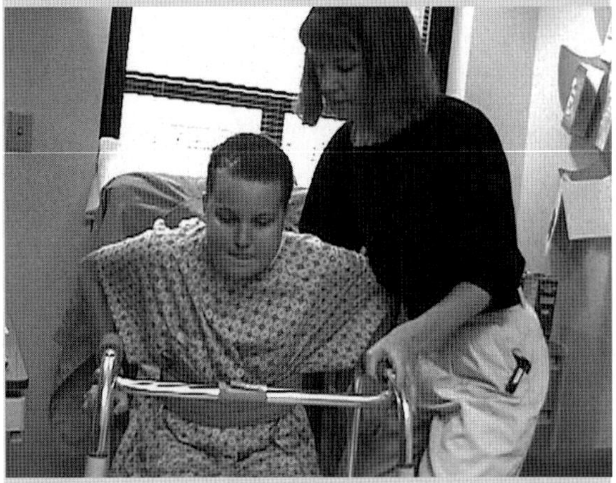

Justin was a resilient, determined kid. After suffering a stroke, he doggedly worked to walk again. He never complained, over nine years of cancer.

had to do it. You had to really watch everything.

His mother did a great job, and he did a fantastic job.

Mothers look at it like, "That's my baby. I don't want you to hurt her or him." Fathers look at it like, "Go, go, go, we've got to get it straightened out."

They misread the spider bite that he had. They misread his meningitis. They misread the stroke. We were leaving the hospital one day, and Justin had just gotten—I think it was the Methotrexate, he laid the seat back in the car and said, "You know something? If they make one more mistake, I'm going to sue the SOBs." He was getting pretty frustrated by it. There is little certainty in medicine.

He had so much stuff—months at a time in the hospital, but he kept pushing. Stroke, meningitis and the (poisonous brown recluse) spider bite were the last two years of his life. He graduated from high school and I said, "What are you going to do now? Go to college?" He said, "I'm going to rest up and make up my mind what to do."

The main thing Justin was interested in was pictures of himself with celebrities, being in the newspaper, and being on television. He loved it. He would have loved this.

In 1997, he relapsed the week before Christmas. I told his mother that I'll go to the hospital with him, you can go back to work and we'll get through it. Initially, we all went back to Children's Hospital. That's the day we met Julia and Steve.

They came in and said these people want to make a film. They became like part of the family. They were very nice people. I think it's because they got so involved with our family.

That day that we went to see (an early version of) the movie, I didn't even think about it that day. I tried my best to keep myself occupied and do other stuff. I went to look at it as a film, not as a story about my son. That's kind of the way I got through it. I did fine.

When Justin died, we were at home. The nurses always thought that he died because we weren't there. I don't know if that was the case. Maybe he was sort of picking his own time.

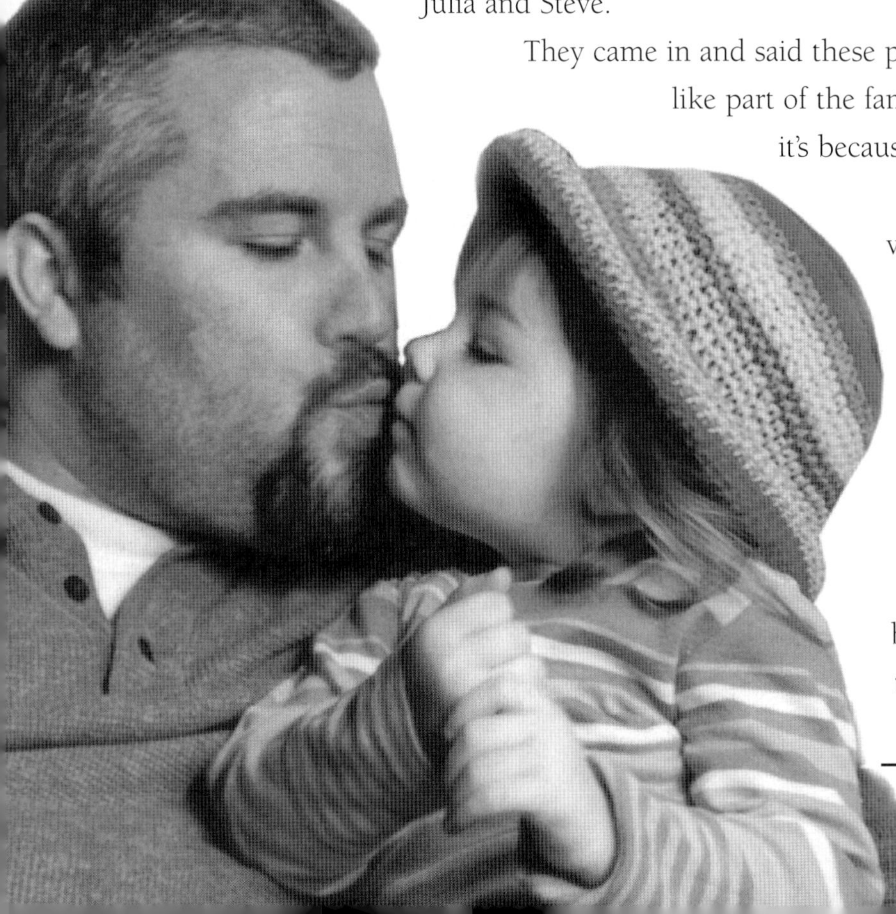

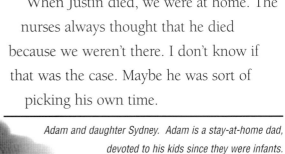

Adam and daughter Sydney. Adam is a stay-at-home dad, devoted to his kids since they were infants.

The doctors, I don't think that they really communicated. The nurses were more in tune with the parents. They were the ones with the hearts. They were the ones to find out who you were dealing with. The residents, Justin called them "half-a-doctors."

My kids are a lot like me. It's a tough group of people with kind of a warped sense of humor where people can laugh about things you normally cannot laugh about. Bad jokes at bad times, doomsday humor, there was a lot of it in the family.

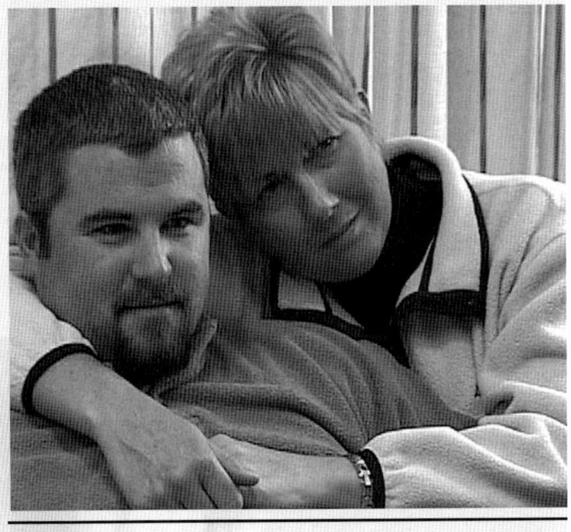

Adam resisted visiting his brother in the hospital. His wife, Shelly, encouraged him to visit and to talk about his long-standing anger and hurt.

My brother lost a four-year-old who got electrocuted in '79, so we have been through trauma in the family over the years. My father died young. I worked for him. He was fifty-six. I went in and talked with my lawyer one day, and he said, "How have you kept from killing yourself?" I said, "I just want to see how it ends." I started over three or four times in my life. Like Justin—we had to teach him how to walk three times in his life.

My brother said that he would go a whole year without thinking of Danny, his little boy. Then all of a sudden, all he'd do is cry. He got electrocuted in '79, so that's twenty-six years? That's kind of a way how it's gotten with me. I would go along and there would be a TV program or something like that and it would hit me.

The kids, Adam and Jennifer, they are doing great. They are really great kids. They had their problems, especially Adam. He's the oldest and he felt the most rejected. That's the way it always is. The healthy kids feel left out because they do not get the same treatment.

With Susan being sick, we are about to get our master's degree in cancer. Yeah, some of these areas of expertise we didn't set out to get.

susanASHCRAFT

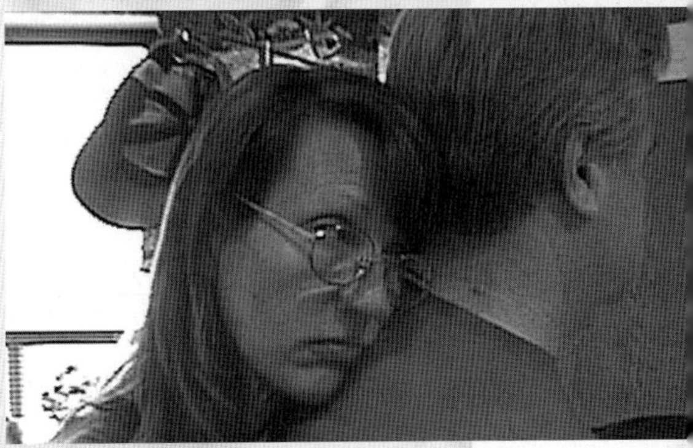

Justin's stepmother, Susan helped Dale and Debbie maintain a round-the-clock-vigil at Children's Hospital for the last six weeks of his life.

Susan Ashcraft is undergoing treatment for thyroid cancer, as she was during the last years of Justin's illness when she helped Debbie and Dale keep vigil at the hospital.

"I hid it while we were going through this with Justin. Dale and I got married in '96, and I already had it then. It is slow growing, but it has gotten progressively worse. Because of what Dale went through with Justin, I think that is what has made him such an understanding husband with my situation. I don't think many men could handle it. Dale is remarkable. *(Susan also suffers from amyloidosis, a condition in which abnormal proteins accumulate in the organs.)*

I got along with Justin great. We had a certain bonding because I have cancer too. I've had it twenty-one years. He was sheltered and more immature than the average 18-year-old. But he was a special kid. He had a great personality.

I didn't want to be in the movie. I felt like there were emotions flying and things coming out of my mouth and I'll regret it later, I know I will. I was the third wheel. I'm hearing and seeing things one way, and a parent is seeing and hearing things another. I just felt like there was that struggle.

By the time this all came down, his doctor decided that she was going to move to Atlanta. She said, "I don't want to leave you not in remission." That started the decision to triple the dose of the Methotrexate. The Methotrexate is what killed Justin. They operated on him on New Year's Eve to find out if there was infection in the brain. That is when they found out there were lesions in the brain as a result of the Methotrexate. That's when they knew that he wasn't going to recover. I feel that's when the support was stopped, and it was a matter of trying to make him comfortable. We had two parents and a half parent here thinking, "What else can we do?" That is where the breakdown was, because his doctor was gone.

One of the big issues that I experienced was that once they realized that Justin wasn't going to survive, they gave up on him. Justin was experiencing pneumonia and hardly being able to breathe. My mom had died just months before, they had suctioned her. We had to say to the doctors, "Can't we suction, Justin?" They said, "If that is what you want us to do." I never felt that they took any initiative to do anything to make Justin better. That bothered me.

Dale, Debbie, and I would share a room with Justin around the clock. February 1st I had to go back to work because I was out of sick days. The end of that week, Dale says, "You need to come over here and relieve me and Debbie so I can go home and sleep in my own bed one night." I went over that night and I stayed with Justin. I remember I went over to him and said, "It's okay, Justin." Believe it or not, he died the next morning while I was there.

Debbie and Dale didn't say, "We left him in your care and he died." It really was true. Believe it or not I felt guilty because I fell asleep. I woke up at five, looked up at the monitor and realized that his blood pressure was going down then, and I didn't know whether I needed to call Debbie and Dale. I wanted them to get rest; I wanted them to sleep. He had gone down once or twice before, but it had bounced back up. So, it was the decision of whether to call them at 5 a.m. and say, "Get yourselves over here." I ended up on the phone at ten to 7 a.m. saying, "You need to get over here immediately." They were both en route, but Justin passed before they both got there.

I lived with that guilt for months. I didn't do my part. I didn't get them there early enough. At the end, I was sure everything was in God's hands and it happened the way God wanted it to happen. I got through that, but it was kind of a traumatic experience for me at the time.

Afterward, I had to be patient because Dale had a lot of healing to do. I know that a part of him went with Justin.

It's portrayed in the movie that Adam didn't really want to be there at the hospital. He didn't want to watch Justin die. He didn't like to go to the hospital. It wasn't because he didn't care; he just didn't want to go through it. He'd been through it for nine years and he didn't want to do it anymore. He has turned into a wonderful father. He does a great job with his children.

adamASHCRAFT

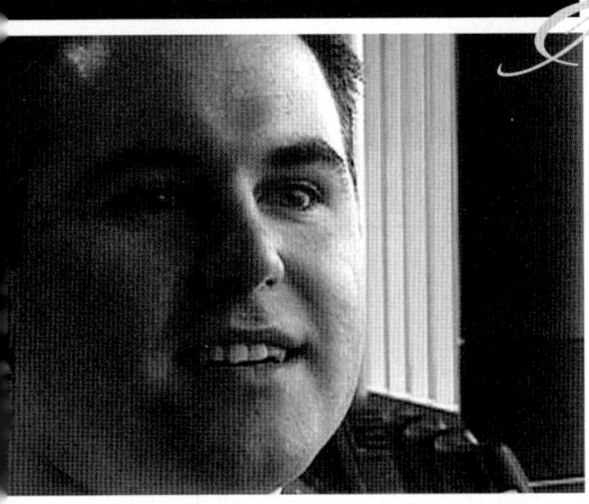

The filmmakers first met Adam Ashcraft at the Cincinnati airport the day Justin and his parents left for treatment in Houston. Adam, recently married, confided that his marriage was in trouble.

Adam, fifteen when his brother Justin was diagnosed, is married and the father of two young children. In the film he talks about the depression that developed during his teen years and shadowed him into adulthood.

When there's an illness like that, the worst thing you can do is not talk about it. Your kids are left to draw their own conclusions, and it scares the hell out of them. We never talked about it in my family. Never. When you're young, you want to know what's going on, but nobody would tell us. We were just left out a lot.

You never did get that sense of "Everything is okay." It was always pins and needles. It's one thing to think it, but to have an adult say, "Everything is okay right now, this is what's going on, it'll be all right," that calming factor never did come in. You're a kid. Your mind wanders. You worry about things.

Your own health is jeopardized, if you're focused on him and you don't pay attention to yourself. Depression slowly creeps in. You tend to surround yourself with people like yourself. All the people I knew, they didn't talk much. I had lived that way for so long. I had thought maybe something was off in the back of my mind, but that's all I knew.

The line was, make like everything's okay and everything will be okay. I always got the feeling that my parents were afraid if they acknowledged it, the wheels would immediately fall off the bus. Something really bad would happen. Have a positive attitude and good things will happen. If we go down the other road, who knows what will happen?

Later on, my wife came along and said, "Wait a minute. This is not a healthy environment." She just kept saying over and over, "There's something wrong, there's something wrong." I could see things were a little rocky and I felt bad. It's hard living with a person that's depressed, it really is.

At first, I'm like, "There's nothing wrong, there's nothing wrong." And then it was "I'll just go to therapy just to shut her up. She just doesn't understand how we work." I always ended up back where I started. It would be good for a couple months to a year, then we'd be having the same conversation again. She got tired of having the same conversation. Then I had kids too, and it's like, gosh, I don't want to pass that along. The kids are going to have enough problems without Dad not being able to function in life.

I still am in therapy now. Three and a half years, every week, every Wednesday at Cincinnati Center for Psychoanalysis. I'd been through a couple (therapists) by trial and error. The whole thing is trial and error. Finding the right therapist, finding the right meds. They don't know what drugs will help you and which drugs will mess you up. The side effects on some of those things are pretty brutal. Most people use Prozac with no problems. I couldn't touch it. It made me delusional. I had the goo-goo-g'joob-I-am-the-walrus syndrome.

Luckily, I started that part before my children came along. I did have what medicines worked for me and which didn't. Then after that, three and a half years later, I'm a heck of a lot better than where I started from.

I'm still affected by the experience. Every time one of my kids gets a cold, the first thing that pops into my mind is, "Oh my gosh, it's something bigger than a cold. This could be cancer." You can't really do that to your children. Most people, when the kid gets a cold, it's a cold. Me, I'm on pins and needles. Little things like that.

Justin's been dead now six years and I'm still going through some of the stuff that I was going through when he was alive. It's like post-traumatic stress. The worst sound in the world is going to a cancer ward and hearing these little kids getting chemo, the screams, those are things you shouldn't hear.

Technology has advanced, they have all these wonderful drugs that can help these kids. But on the mental side of it, it's still like the 1940s for these kids. To see kids go through that and not have some kind of problems or issues is ridiculous. On the mental side, there are a lot of problems there that haven't been addressed. A lot of people don't think about that. They can make your kid healthy, but mentally, he's a mess. People think you can throw 'em a pill, slap 'em on the bottom, and they're well. Unfortunately, it doesn't work like that.

Justin was not as mature as kids his age. A lot of that had to do with the drugs; they slowed him down mentally. It just took a couple of years off of him. Then on top of that, the social situation, it's isolating for everyone around, for the children and for the families. All your attention is on this ailment, and friends don't like to hang out with that stuff, his friends or your friends. Who likes to talk about cancer with children?

Justin's case was even worse because he was in and out of school; it was hard. Like mom said, no dance, no prom. I saw that and at the end of his life he was really depressed, probably the last year and a half. I could tell because he had the same symptoms I did. You can tell things are going to be hard and difficult (medically) and the last thing you want is for the kid to be depressed. You know, sleep all day, up all night. That bothered me a lot.

(The movie depicts the struggle of Justin's family to decide when to cease treatment after doctors said he would not recover.)

We'd gone through it for such a long time that in the back of your mind you're like, "God, he's pulled out of so many things like this. There is a possibility (of survival)." It was tough just because a lot of our life was cancer. Then it was coming to an end. So what do we do? How does it end?

Unfortunately with Justin, the end was worse than I think any of us had ever thought or imagined it would have been for him. That whole time, I couldn't really even talk to him in his last moments. There's only a couple things in life I regret and that's one of them. You don't get a do-over on that. At the end of his life, I didn't get a chance to talk to him and tell him what he really meant to me and express how much I loved him.

That's why you've got to talk to your children. It's not a bad thing. It's hard, but it has to be done. It's not an option.

It would be nice to have at least a second layer behind you, a safety net, somebody to turn to you and say, "Hey, what's going on?" Steve and Julia were the first people that came up to me and asked me the question. "What's going on, Adam? What's really happening?" That's all it took. After that, a lot of things really changed for me. It was them saying, "It's okay to talk about this. We're not going to judge you. We know things are crappy. We'd like to hear it." That was probably one of the most important moments in my life, running into those two. That, on top of meeting my wife; it was all about the same time.

Jennifer was 13 when Justin was diagnosed. I'm sure it was tough. That's the thing, I had another sibling and we never did talk about it. We've talked about it now.

The same relationship I had with my brother, I have with my sister. Lately, it's a lot better than it was. It's not anywhere near normal, but probably about as normal as it's going be.

(Adam attended the Sundance Film Festival with his parents and sister.)

I only saw my dad cry about it twice—once when Justin was diagnosed and once when he was getting ready to die. But at the film festival, everybody was just in tears. You watch the film and you could see everybody handled it the best way they knew how to.

There's something about being a theater with 200, 300 people and there's not a dry eye in the house, everyone's crying. Then to realize why, because of what's going on up on the screen, it's extremely powerful. At first at the festival it was overwhelming, but now that all that's past and I'm back to my normal stuff, it makes you appreciate what was actually on the screen and the impact it possibly could have on other people.

I'm looking at this film and it seems like a lifetime ago. It transports you back to the time, and I'm thinking, "Man, I was one messed-up fella." I was the quiet one; those aren't the ones who get the help or attention they need. I slipped through the cracks, both educationally and emotionally. I never did graduate from high school; it drives me nuts to this day.

That's the neat thing about Sundance—it's not just fans of film; you get the whole business side too. You've got executives and buyers and even artists themselves. There was another documentary gentleman there and he's in tears. You knew it was special just by listening to the regular people in the audience.

At the last screening, one gentleman was about my age and he said how it hit home with him because his brother had cancer too about the same age, and he survived and he's going to be a doctor now. He said, "Thank you, because I went through the same thing." He's up there crying while saying this. It was overwhelming. I don't usually get that in my stay-at-home father routine.

That kind of emotion from an audience, I just didn't expect it. Plus, everybody stayed for the whole thing. Who the hell is going to sit through three hours and 45 minutes of this film? Who wants to go see a film about kids with cancer? There's no way you could get that many people to stay through the whole thing if it's just horrible children-with-cancer stuff. That's the nice thing about the film. It's well balanced.

I was just amazed at my parents, because I'm sure they didn't think it was going to be anything like this. It seems weird too—they didn't want to talk much with us; why would they want to do a documentary? When you see the interviews with my parents and Jennifer, this is the first time I'm hearing these things, their thoughts, their ideas, what's going on in their heads.

For a while after Justin died and Steve and Julia would pop in, following up, I'd think, "Is this thing ever going to be done? I'm done with all this, I want to get on with my life. Quit showing up and asking all these questions." Now, I'm extremely grateful. The work is just unbelievable.

I thought it was going to be this little obscure thing no one was ever going to see. I'm thinking, documentary filmmakers from Yellow Springs, okay, right, going to be a bunch of hippies with a video camera. Then you look at the finished product and you're just blown away.

We got to meet all the editors, a lot of people involved with the film. They surrounded themselves with excellent people. A lot of the editors would come up and say, "Thank you, it was an honor to work on this film and get to know you through this film." I felt really bad because I could only get out two lines because I was going to cry every time they came up. I called them later when I got home. You realize the sacrifices they made. That's hard, watching it over and over again. Sure it's a job, but that's tough. Unbelievable people involved with this film.

As painful as it was to watch, I still got to see my brother on the screen. A lot of people don't get that opportunity. It was hard, but it was nice to see him up there, to see the effect he had and all the other kids had on all these people.

jenniferASHCRAFT

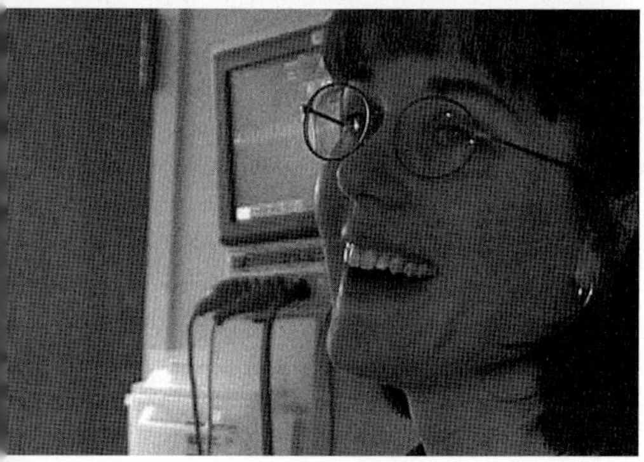

Justin's older sister, Jennifer, was jealous of the attention showered on him in the early years of his illness. In time, they became close, particularly after she donated her bone marrow for his treatment.

(Justin's only sister is now a mother herself.)

I was only twelve when he was diagnosed; it's hard for a twelve-year-old kid. When your parents are like, "Okay, sorry we don't have time for you anymore; we'll see ya later," I was very jealous. Probably like the first two years. When you're twelve, you don't understand.

I remember they were supposed to pick me up at school, not being there, Adam riding up on his ten-speed saying, "Hey, Mom had to take Justin to the doctor," and I was like, "Great, that means I have to walk home from school."

I got home and I was like "Where are they?" Things were not right. They walked in the door and the look on their faces was like they were just run over by a truck. Poor Justin was so small. I remember him sitting in a chair and they took us back in a bedroom and told us, "Justin's really sick. He has leukemia, which is cancer." I remember my father crying; I don't remember Mom crying. I can remember them saying, "You're going to have to stay at your aunt and uncle's for a while because we need to be with Justin."

I didn't really have anybody to talk to. I remember getting out the encyclopedia to find out what leukemia was.

I felt abandoned. I felt pushed to the side, like it was going to be like that forever. I didn't really understand how he was going to get out of the hospital or if he even was, if he was going to survive. Because everyone was crying and saying Justin might die. And I was like, "Am I going to have to live with my aunt and uncle forever?" They didn't really explain to us. But they were shocked and overwhelmed like everyone else.

I know that was the last thing they were thinking about was their other two children. Looking back on it now I know that, but at the time—that's why parents really need to sit down and explain what's going on with their other children when they're as young as we were. Maybe that would help.

The older I got, I never had any resentment. I knew the seriousness of the situation and if they could not be there, I knew why. I knew that Justin needed them more than I did. I got mature at a very young age because of this life situation I was thrown into.

With me and Justin it was just (she makes a snarling nose and holds her hands up like claws) all the time. Just such conflicting personalities. But he's my little brother. Justin and I were close even though we had different viewpoints on every single thing in life. With his leukemia, with me being his bone marrow donor, we always had a special closeness that only two siblings, I think, could share.

I think about him daily, I'd say. As time goes on, the pain gets a little better. But, every day, I think about him.

I think about things we used to do together, how silly we'd get. I'd rather not remember him lying there in the hospital bed, watching that stupid monitor. I don't like to think about the last few months of his life because it was so bad. I try not to think about too much of the hospital because that just wasn't Justin.

When they put him in ICU, I was at work, I got a call saying, "He's not doing so well, you need to get there," and that was the first time we all sort of panicked. And he was still conscious at that time, and he was looking at me like, "Help me; I can't do anything; what's wrong?" And when everyone was out of the room talking, I said, "Justin, it's going be okay. Just sit back and try to breathe. Calm down and everything's going to be all right." I think at that time he tried to shut his eyes. I knew that there wasn't any getting better from there; it was only going to get worse.

Actually, his last word was to me. I came into the room and said, "Hi Justin." He mumbled, "Hi," and that was the last time he ever spoke to anybody.

(At the hospital) Adam made the comment, "Isn't enough enough?" and Mom got very upset with that. I think we all realized it, but when you're a parent, any ounce of hope that anyone gives you, you're going to go with it. If he died of the leukemia she would have been like, "Well, why didn't I do the triple? That may have helped him." Any way you went, it would have been a horrible situation.

They did what they thought was going to help him. No way could anyone have ever known what would happen. They say the most horrifying death is of your child. I don't think there's anything you can ever say to anyone to make them get over such a horrifying thing. There's nothing anyone could say to me. Nobody knows until you go through it, until you experience the pain, the loss, there's nothing anybody could say.

The first week, after he died, I stayed here and watched the dogs while Mom went to Florida, and that was just weird. I swear there were weird things going on in this house. You can feel his presence so much when you walk down the stairs. Anywhere else in the house, it's fine, but once you walk down the steps and especially when you hit his room, you're like, "Oh God, he's here."

I remember Mom making tea one day and getting ready to call down the steps for Justin to down there anymore." That's the hardest. That and holidays. Christmas especially, because I spent his last Christmas dinner feeding my brother. And that's the only memory that I really dwell on, the negative memory. To have to cut up my brother's food and have to feed him with his little cup and straw.

I'm comfortable with his death. Nobody's comfortable with the way he died but me. Which is weird. Because I thought he was just kind of peaceful and he waited for his time and did it on his terms. No one was around. Justin wouldn't have it any other way but his way. I think it was horrible, the way he was overdosed. But blaming the doctors is just—they did what they thought they could do to help him. The outcome was more than anyone could have expected; but I think that he died a pretty peaceful death.

In order to bring closure and peace within yourself, you have to talk about things. You have to realize that everything happens for a reason. Sure, Justin had a horrifying disease, but he did bring a lot of joy into a lot of people's lives. He brought a lot of good, and even in the medical field, they made a lot of advances because of Justin.

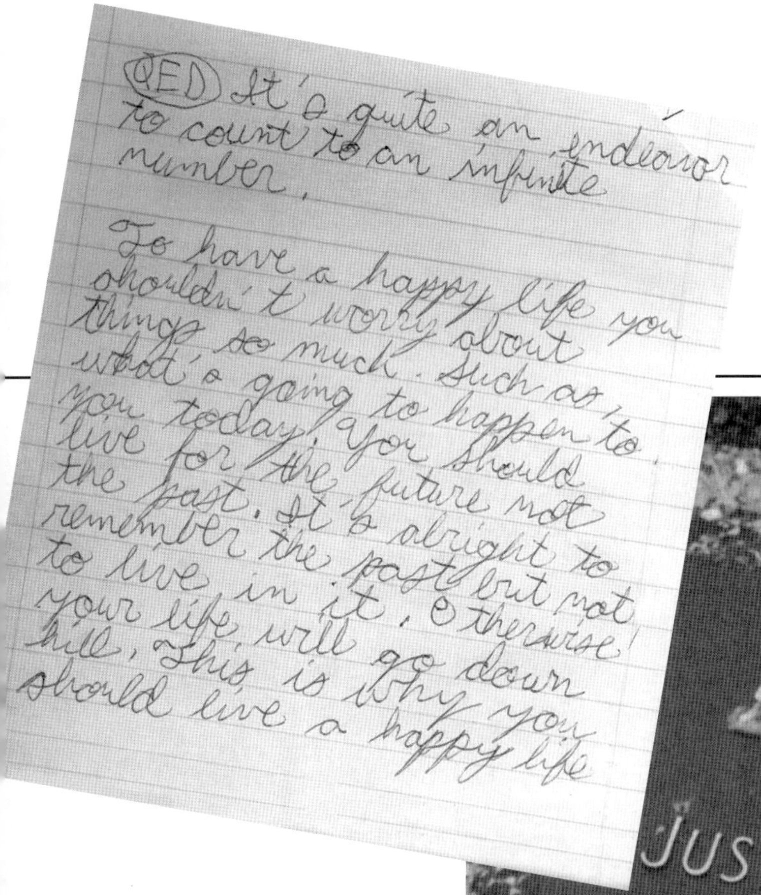
QED It's quite an endeavor to count to an infinite number.

To have a happy life you shouldn't worry about things so much. Such as, what's going to happen to you today. You should live for the future not the past. It's alright to remember the past but not to live in it. Otherwise your life will go down hill. This is why you should live a happy life

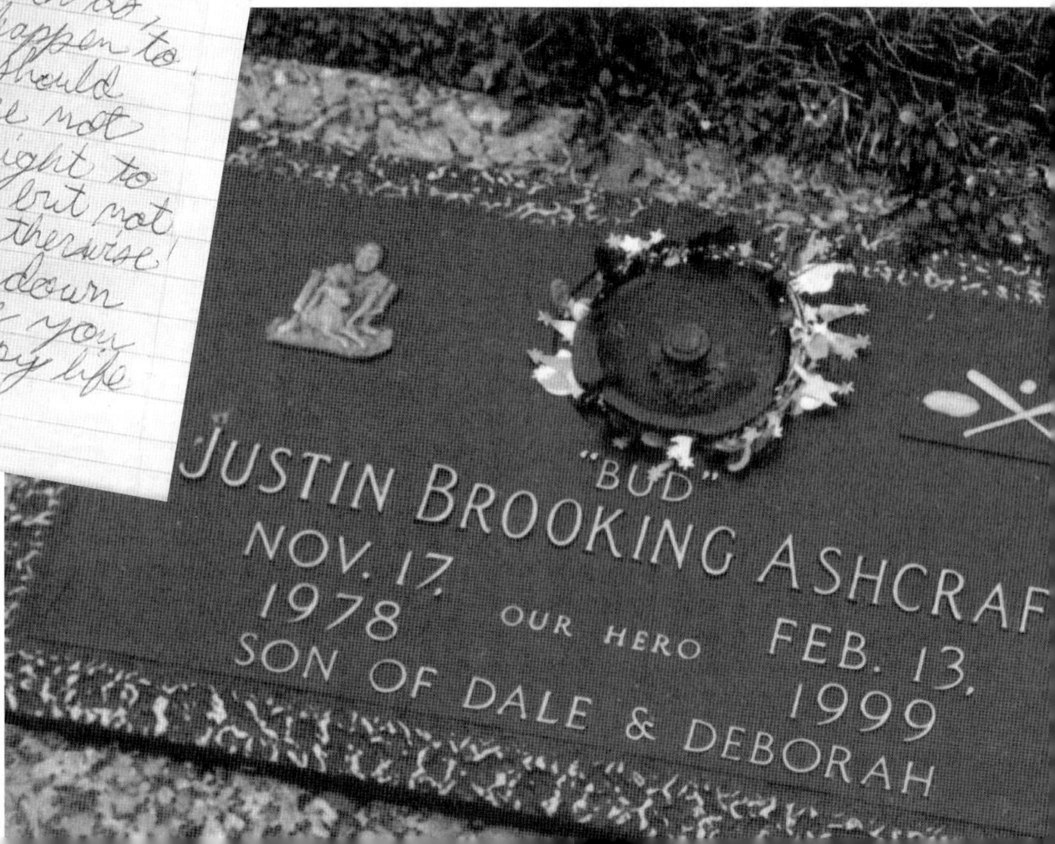

Filmmakers' Journal

Julia: It was near Christmas, and we were in the clinic. We heard the Ashcrafts were there and someone from the hospital said, "They're in the room right now with their doctor. Just go in, introduce yourself, get started."

Steven: We realized they were having a really serious meeting, and that we shouldn't start with us talking, but by shooting.

Julia: So we went in and started shooting almost immediately. I'm pretty sure we got nods from them. We realized quickly it was a very somber room. Important decision-making was going on, Justin had relapsed, his cancer had come back, and the family was trying to decide what to do.

But once they talked over the options, and the decision was made, the room pretty much erupted into back-and-forth banter, mainly between Dale and Justin. The room quickly broke into hilarity, really.

None of this is in the film, but once the joking started, and Dr. Claire Mazewski kept examining Justin, they were giving him a razzing about his new glasses, about how scary it was that Justin now had his temp driver's permit. Dr. Claire said, "Could you send us all an e-mail before you get on the highway, so we all know to stay off the road?" They teased him about how his sister dressed him up in her clothing. That's how we were introduced to the Ashcrafts' biting humor.

Steven: They would make jokes that were kind of shocking. Like when someone at the hospital would offer Justin a living will form, his dad would say, "Does that mean I get the baseball cards?" Dale made jokes about going on the "Justin Ashcraft Memorial Cruise" with Justin's money after he was gone. To someone just walking in the room, the stuff they said would raise your eyebrows. But Justin threw it back as good as he got it, and that was one of their ways of dealing with the madness of ten years of fighting cancer. They were like the most battle-hardened troops of a war. The jokes helped them through.

Julia: They seemed to have an endless supply of good, biting humor. But then Adam would say, later on, that these jokes got in the way of being open with each other to talk about the hard stuff.

I liked Debbie right away. I think we struck up a bond, a bit. The two moms. Debbie and I had long phone conversations between shooting.

Steven: The Ashcrafts were immediately warm and open to us. We didn't know at the time that they were media veterans, because Bud (Justin) had done so many interviews and TV news segments. So they were pretty relaxed around us immediately. We later found out that Debbie and Dale were cool with this because Justin wanted us around. He liked the cameras and the attention.

At first, Dale intimidated me. Here's this big, square-jawed, rock-ribbed guy—clearly not the kind of guy you see running around in our little hippie town of Yellow Springs. He wasn't always a man of many words, so I would get nervous about what he was thinking. But he's a deeply caring man, a real sensitive guy, though I'm not sure he'd want me to say that.

Julia: Justin and his family were very relaxed, very open, they seemed to want to include us in everything. They were fun to be around.

Steven: They had such big personalities.

Julia: Once we got to know Jennifer and Adam, a lot more became clear, to us, about this family. Jennifer was often present, but seldom heard. To me, she was very protective of her mother and through the years had learned how to make herself undemanding—a supportive, undemanding presence. By contrast, Adam felt a lot of anger and fear. He drew away from the family, and had a lot to say to us. He really helped us understand how his family works. I started referring to him as the "truth teller."

Steven: There's one incident that for me sums up how crazy their situation was. Here's Justin, fighting cancer for years and years. One time when he was a teenager, he got a chance to go to a cancer camp to hang out with other survivors. They go on a hike in the woods, and Justin sees a cobweb. Being the ornery kid he is, he puts his hand through the cobweb. And he gets bit by a spider. A rare, poisonous spider, called a brown recluse. It's like the second deadliest spider after the black widow. And he nearly dies, and ends up in the hospital for weeks. Because he got to go to cancer camp. To me, that sums up the level of absurdity these folks lived with.

Julia: It really astounded me how Debbie would go toe-to-toe with the doctors, and seemed to really understand all the complicated treatments, decisions, chemos, side effects. Everything. She read a lot. She had a great memory. All with a high school education. She was always smiling, always the solid advocate for Justin.

Julia: Gramma (Debbie's mother) was a hoot.

Steven: She was always flirting with me! Saying stuff like "This ol' gal's still got it, honey."

Julia: She was angry a lot of the time, too.

Steven: Grammas speak their mind. Once you get your gramma membership card, you get to be really blunt with everyone. At least that's true for all the grammas I know.

I would say they understood, all of them, that they had different roles to play, and that actually for a lot of families that might be a good way to do it. Like a team—you have different people in different roles.

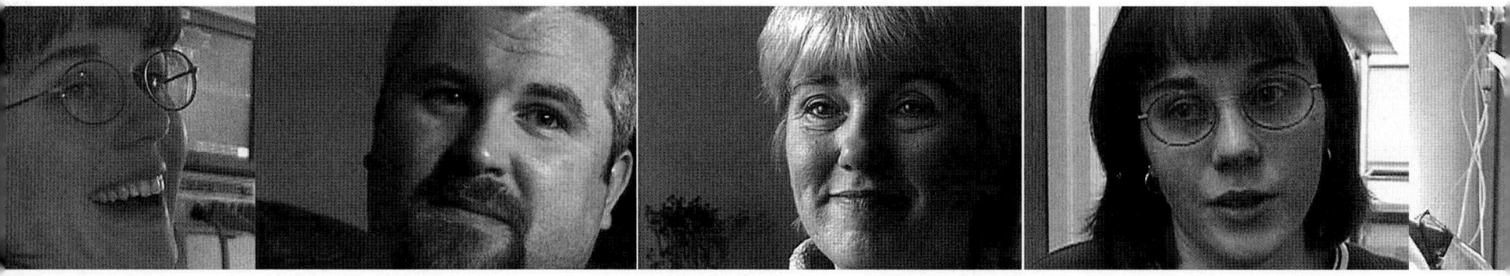

Julia: Deb and Susan, Dale's new wife, got along beautifully. Susan was a very level-headed presence. The Ashcrafts encompassed a huge extended family; there were always brothers and sisters of Dale on hand whenever needed, and Justin had close cousins he spent time with. It was painful to us to have to cut them out of the film for length.

Steven: Justin's cousins speak so movingly about how they felt about Justin's situation, how it upset them that he never got to do the stuff a normal teenager should do. Like something as simple as driving. I hope we can put this stuff on the DVD.

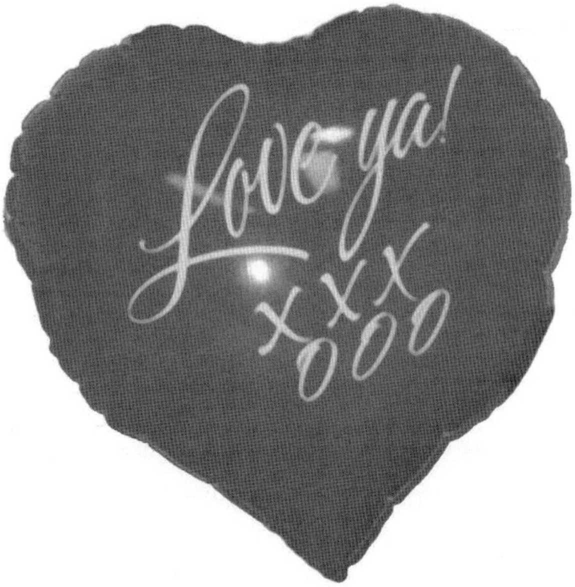

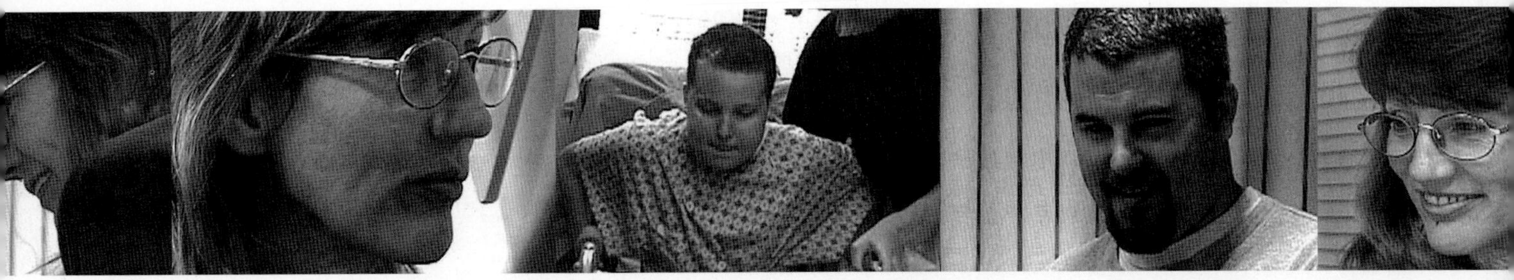

Chapter 2

Jennifer Moone

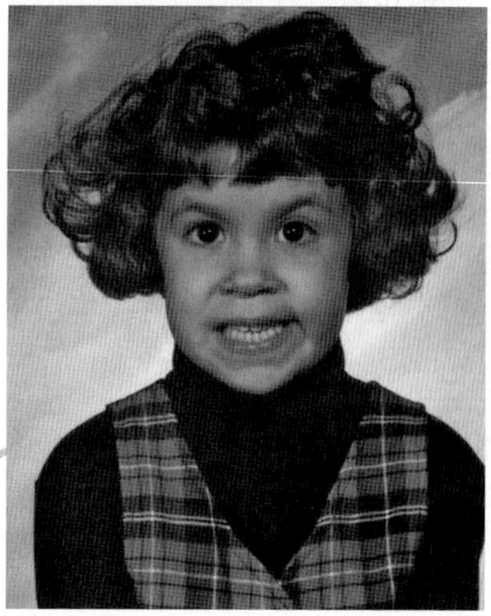

Jen's Kindergarten picture

jennifer&natalie

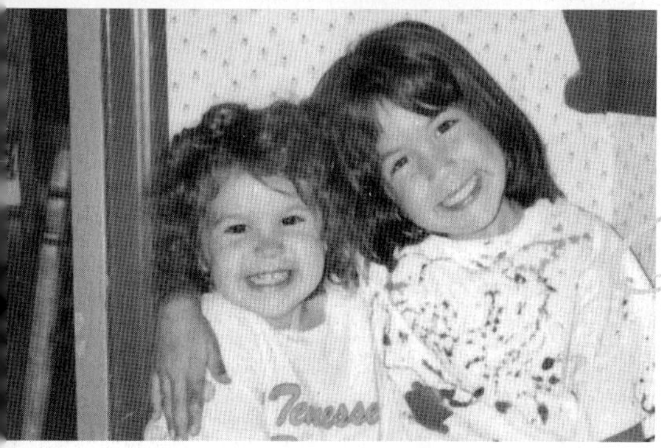

Jen and her older sister Natalie, before leukemia struck.

Jennifer was diagnosed shortly before the family moved from Columbus to Cincinnati, where Frank Moone had a new job. Beth Moone quit her full-time job to look after Jennifer and her older daughter Natalie while Jennifer was being treated.

Jen was five. It was in the fall of 1996, I guess, and she started having ear infections again. She had tubes in her ears, but she started getting fevers with the ear infections, which is kind of unusual, but yet, nothing alarming. Then January of 1997, she started getting lethargic, just not herself, tired, taking naps. She's always been a nap person, but still—she started getting one ear infection after another.

We knew she was really sick for about four months. We knew something was wrong. We kept taking her to the pediatrician and they would keep sending us home. "It's a virus. Go home. She's fine." We'd say, "No, wait a minute. Nobody in our home has a virus. She doesn't have any symptoms of a virus other than a fever."

When we finally got the appointment with Children's (in Columbus), we met with the chief of hematology and oncology. He said, "Guys, you aren't thinking that this is something serious are you?" We said, "Yeah, we think there is."

He says, "Well, we can do a test. We can do a bone marrow test if you think that you would feel more comfortable with that. It's kind of painful." Frank and I are like, "Yes, we need to find out." So he did the procedure and he told me,

"Folks, go home." I remember that this was the day after Mother's Day. She was sick on Mother's Day with a slight fever.

So we were home. She wasn't feeling well and had a fever that day. She was sitting on this chair with my husband in the family room, and I got the call two hours later. The doctor was shocked. Here he had just sent the parents home two hours prior saying, "It's nothing, it's very minor." Jennifer did not present a typical diagnosis. She wasn't bleeding. She wasn't bruising, but still, we knew something was wrong. He said, "She has leukemia. You need to come back downtown to the hospital."

I just remember that car ride. I was in so much shock sitting in his office. He said to me, "Do you work full time?" I said, "Yes." He said, "Well, you are probably going to have to take a leave of absence." I said, "What?" He said, "She's going to be in treatment. Where do you work?" I said, "The attorney general's office." He said, "Oh, my son is assistant attorney general in Massachusetts." I was thinking, *I don't care! You just told me that my daughter has cancer! I don't care!*

Jen was just scared. She didn't feel good. She was so tired. We really tried to keep it together for her. You just have to do that for kids, you know? She would do the treatment and go through all this and have a smile on her face. I cried a lot, but tried not to in front of her.

It was so hard for me, the first week, when she was in the hospital in Columbus (where the family still lived) and her pediatrician was in China, the one that had seen her, and her partner would come in, and it was really hard for me to be civil to her. Not only did they miss it, but they just kept dismissing me. They just didn't listen to me as a parent.

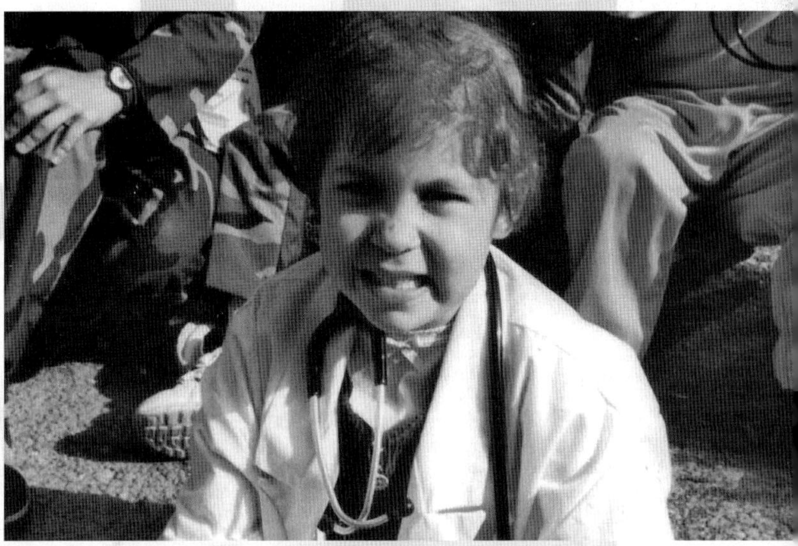

Jen loved to play doctor.

And I really think that you know. If your child is just laying around all the time, you know. You know it's not normal.

We didn't know anything about leukemia. At that point you are even so shocked to hear any statistics or anything about it that it just kind of goes in one ear and out the other. You can't absorb all that at once. You are just not ready for everything at that point.

I just remember all the specialists coming in and talking to us about clinical trials, and giving us all these pamphlets that we had to read. At night she'd be sleeping, and I'd be reading all these documents, trying to figure them out. My sister and my friend who was a nurse sat in when the doctor talked to us, explained the treatment, talked about the drug study, do you want her in a clinical trial, to figure out what we're going to do.

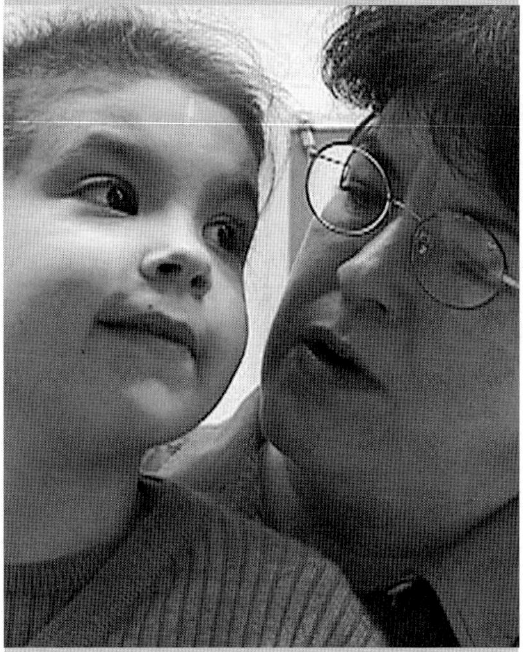

Jennifer talks with her mom, Beth. Jen remembers exactly how many spinal taps she has had—eight so far.

You make a decision about whether you want to put your child in a study, and you're in such shock, and you have a lot of hesitation about whether you're making the right decision. You listen to the doctors, and they're telling you what you should do, and you're just in a daze. You're like, "Yes" and "No" and later you think about it. But you have to make a lot of decisions right away, and it's hard.

When the nurses came in that first week and said, "This is what you have to do with this shot." I mean, I had never—what person who is not in the medical field has ever given someone a shot? Unless, you know, a diabetic. So my hands were shaking, and here I am doing this on my child and thinking, *Am I going to hurt her?*

She loves to be involved in the therapy. And at Childrens' in Cincinnati they're so good about explaining everything. All of her baby dolls had C-lines or spinal taps.

You can't plan much. So it's true; the good days, you get out there, you have fun. The bad days, you don't. But it makes you appreciate them. You appreciate the simple things, like walking to Graeter's to get ice cream.

She was so good about going through what she had to go through, that I couldn't let myself get down. She was just strong, strong. She never complained at all about this illness. Until she went through the second intensification, where she was so sick with the spinal headache, she said, "Mom I don't like having leukemia."

Frank would leave and go to work every day. He had to. I was there. I was there for the clinic visits. And there's times when as a mom, or whoever the caregiver is—not that I was jealous, but I was like, "You can go to work, but I'm here."

Then there were those times when he was able to step in when I wasn't. He would hold her hand in the clinic while I would stand back in the hallway because I had just fallen apart. And you know, the respect that I had for him, I would be like, how could he do that? But, you know, thank God, because I can't. The time that she was so dehydrated that she couldn't even sit up in the chair, and I got in there, and the nurses are all rushing around with the IVs; I had a really hard time with that. I don't know where Frank pulled his inner strength from, but he did it.

Jennifer clings to her mother right after a spinal tap.

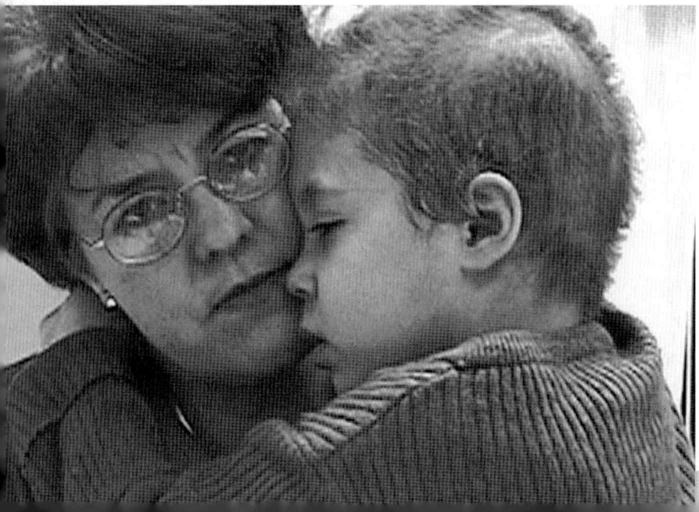

I worked in Columbus (Ohio) for eighteen years. I never went back to work in that office. Three months later, when she was kind of stable, I went up to Columbus and cleaned out my office. It was huge staying home since I hadn't for years, especially staying home with a sick child.

We were always a two-income family with two children *(before Jennifer's illness, Beth worked as an insurance fraud investigator for the Ohio attorney general's office).* We were facing our child's illness. We were also faced with, "Oh, my gosh, now we are losing a whole income." However, in my office they had a program where, if you had so many vacation hours built up, that you could donate those to a co-worker in need. My husband also worked in the attorney general's office. They donated over a year's time for me. Oh, my Lord. So for a whole year, I got a paycheck. At least for a year, that was not a burden on us at that point. That was nice.

We had health insurance, but still we had so many issues with billing and incorrect billing. You are trying to go through this ordeal, and you are getting bills in the mail. I finally got a contact at the hospital so that if I had a question I could call that person. I wasn't put on hold, I wasn't disconnected. I think they now have a place like that to support families, because you do not need that extra stress.

I had to fight so hard in getting them to diagnose her. The nurses were so condescending to me. They would come in and say, "What's going on?" I would ask, "Will you please look back in her chart?" They wouldn't look backwards at what had transpired in her history. Then, I'm in the hospital with the treatments, and I'm fighting and fighting and fighting. Now, she has some learning disabilities, and I'm fighting again. So I think it has made me be a stronger advocate. I am more vocal because of it.

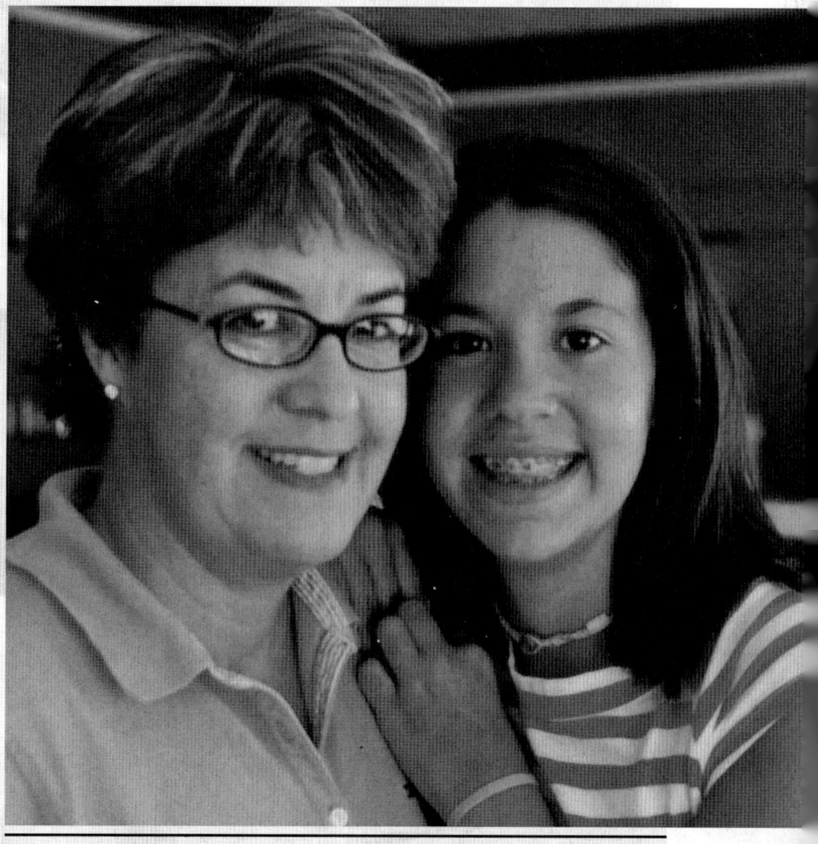

Beth and Jen

She went through so much. I'm not going to let a school system bring her down. She has a learning disability, but she is so motivated. I think it's because of the Methotrexate. She has tutoring every day. She goes to regular classes, but she has a lot of modifications in her work.

She has short-term memory loss, and she has a visual deficiency in structure. All these standardized tests, she can read the question, but when she goes to fill in the bubble, her marks don't line up. That could have been there before, but she was so little. She missed a lot of kindergarten. She missed four months of first grade. There was a lot where she was behind. Math is hard. She doesn't see a shape the way we see it. She has found that it is amazing what she can do with her colored pencils. She's studying for a map test. If she outlines Syria in yellow and Libya in purple, then she can tell the difference. If she doesn't and it's all in pencil or pen, then everything kind of looks the same to her. She really works hard.

I tend to want to be so protective. I'll think, everything she went through, and I'll get emotional. Why does she have to go through anything else? And I know that that's just life. Everybody has their crosses to bear. That's why I have to be such an advocate for her. It's sometimes overwhelming. I wish I could just say, "Heck with it," you know? She's fine, she'll be fine; she might struggle a little bit, but she'll be fine. She'll be an average student, and she might struggle a little bit, but she'll be fine. No! That's not what she wants. And that's not what I want for her.

We heard about the movie when the nurse practitioner said there was a documentary that was going to be proposed. Would we be willing to talk to Julia Reichert and Steve Bognar about participating in this documentary? We talked to them. At the time I didn't realize what it was going to be, how extensive. I didn't realize it for years, because I didn't have any experience working in film. I had no idea that it would be so time-consuming for them. They were around. We didn't know the extent of things that were going to happen. The way they presented it, they didn't know for sure what kind of attention the documentary was going to get. They didn't know whether it would be used for teaching purposes or what it would be exactly used for. I thought if it could help others, why not? Jennifer was so little it didn't matter to her about the cameras being around. She was herself. I think it affects adults more.

Sometimes I would say, "You know, this is kind of a hard time." They were kind and would leave. It was harder after she finished treatment. They would want to attend some of her activities. That's when Jennifer was vocal enough to say, "Mom, I really don't want them around. I really want to be just a normal kid right now. I don't want that attention." I talked to Julia. She understood and backed off. She said, "No problem."

Watching the film, it's difficult for my husband, because I was kind of a main caregiver for her in terms of taking her to the clinic. Other than the first spinal tap, Frank could never go in there. He couldn't handle that procedure. So that's in the film, and he's watching the spinal tap. It's very difficult.

It's also difficult what those other families are going through. Some of their children died. We wanted to see it ahead of time so we can figure out how to prepare Jennifer about it. She's going to relive it. A lot of it she forgets. Is she going to be upset watching, with what has happened to the other two children, especially because they had the same type of leukemia that she had? One little girl looks so much like Jennifer that my oldest thought that it was Jennifer.

There's also parts in the film where I'm talking about how I didn't know if she was going to make it. That's going to be hard, but there are also some very positive scenes. I love it at the end where she's on the deck and she's talking about how she's excited about being in swim team.

I love the interview with my husband where he says I'm the one who had to change my life, Jennifer couldn't have done it without me, he knew I was special the day he married me. I was thinking, "Wow, I wish he told me that when we were going through this!" There were times when I thought, "Yeah, he gets to leave." I knew that was the place where I wanted to be, but it's difficult on a relationship, a child's illness like that.

Natalie, she never really showed her emotion. Everybody thought that was really strange, but that's kind of the way she is. We knew she was real sensitive to it. Every time she would get sick, she told us—now, after the fact—that she was afraid she was getting leukemia. She was kind of easing into the transition of a new school system also, trying to make new friends.

For the first two years she kind of struggled in school. For two years we had to focus on Jennifer. Trips were planned and cancelled; that was kind of hard for Natalie. Plus, she was worried about her little sister. We really tried to split up so Frank would take Natalie on special things and I would have Jennifer. We didn't want her to feel left out. I think she thought that we moved here because of Jennifer. That's not true. We didn't move here because it's a better hospital. She kind of made that up.

Jen was showered with gifts. And maybe half the people were conscientious enough to get something for Natalie too.

It was definitely stressful. There were a lot of nights where we'd have to take off and go to the emergency room. We were fortunate enough to have wonderful neighbors down the street. I could call Lori and say, "Can you take Natalie?" She would make sure she would get to school and did her homework. Natalie is a really good athlete. Basketball is her sport. Frank would travel with her and go places. I think that was a good thing for her. She had something that was holding her attention in a positive way.

Jennifer has had a couple of health scares in the past few years, like pneumonia. I could tell with Natalie's reaction that it really scares her, more so than "My brother or sister has a cold." She has that awareness. I think she also lives life to the fullest too. They always say if you have cancer and you are a survivor, you always live each day. I think that even as a sibling she thinks, *I'm lucky, she's lucky, I'm going to make the most of my life.*

I do think it changed my priorities. When I decided that I needed to go back to work, I tried to go back to work for eight months. I realized that I couldn't do that. I didn't have enough time to spend with my kids. So I asked them if I could work part-time. It's perfect.

We do volunteer with the Leukemia and Lymphoma Society. The girls do all kinds of things in the summer. Jennifer's a hero for their Team in Training program.

People look at Jen and they'll go, "Gosh, isn't it amazing to think of what happened to her, and look at her now." That's what everybody says: "Look at her now." And she has so many friends. I used to look at her in the playground, and she didn't have any friends. She'd be sitting by herself reading a book or something. And now she has tons of friends. I mean, she has tons of friends. Somebody is always calling, and the kids love her.

It makes her feel really sad to think about the kids who aren't making it. I have to watch about volunteering for the Leukemia Society, because that's really starting to bother her. And they're finding that that's more of an issue with females. They tend to feel survivorship guilt. Little girls. Because so many kids are not making it.

With her cancer behind her, Jen works hard to manage its late effects, while living a normal life.

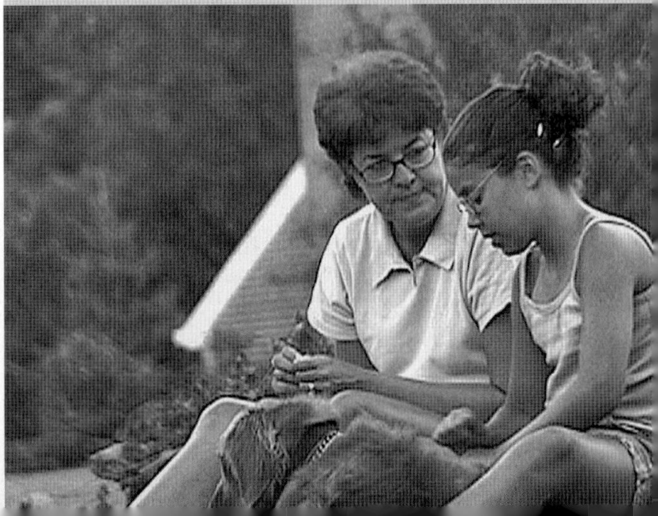

I gave in to her a little bit more than I normally would. I asked myself, would I do this if she wasn't sick? You know, I think I gave in more to my kids when I was a working mom, because I wasn't around. I've gained more patience, definitely, since I've been at home. I notice more. They've learned more what my limits are.

There's been a lot of friends who came up to me and said, "I could never have done this," and I'm like, "Yes you can." You have to. I mean, how can you not? You find it in yourself. To me, you have no choice.

I'm thinking more now of what I went through. I was so involved, with her treatment, moving her, new schools, new job for Frank. I just did it.

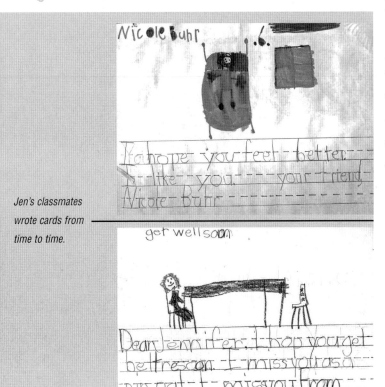

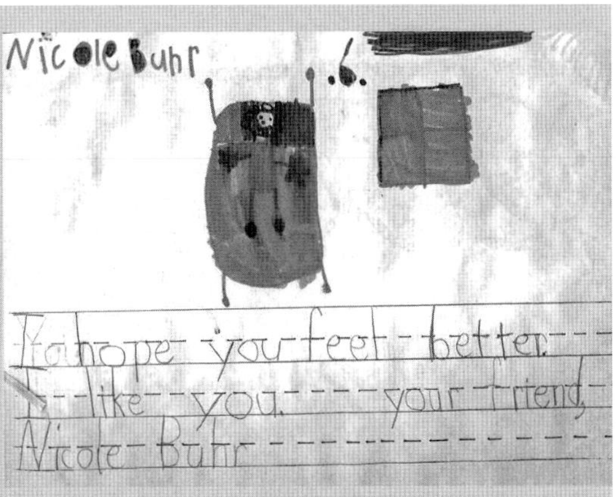

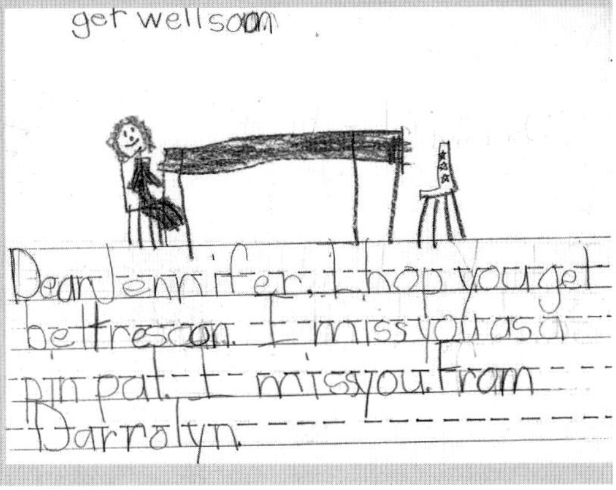

Jen's classmates wrote cards from time to time.

The hardest part is seeing your child so sick. And thinking how this is not fair. Being angry. Thinking, *What have they done?* And just kind of being angry at things. And you look back at your life before that and think, *Gosh, life was good.* Your life was so good (laughs). Why were we ever complaining?

It forced me to slow down. And that's what I needed to do. My life was out of control. I was trying to be the perfect mother, the perfect employee. I was in a position where I was a supervisor; I had fifteen people I was supervising. I had a boss who was kind of hard to get along with. So I was trying to be perfect there. And have the perfect home. Well, you can't do that. And so it was almost like you need to adjust things a little bit and slow down.

And our life's better. With Frank and me, he comes home, we're just not as stressed. I used to yell. I know I did. I just didn't have any patience. You know, I'd get home, I'd have paperwork, and I'd be working with them, and I don't know how I did it.

It seemed like we never had enough time. We'd work, we'd come home, it would be six o'clock, we'd be fixing dinner, we'd want to go to the park, but we had homework, so we tried to get in that quality time, but we often couldn't do it. Then I traveled quite a bit with my job, so Frank would be there. We're pretty equal in parenting, equal in the chores we had to do.

I feel more caring. I feel like I was living before, but not really living, I feel like I'm just more conscious of what's really important. The things I thought were important, they mean nothing.

And maybe that is why, because of what we have been through, I am not a worrier anymore. If something happens we will deal with it, but I am definitely going to live each day to the fullest, and that stayed with me, and if it creeps away, I bring it back.

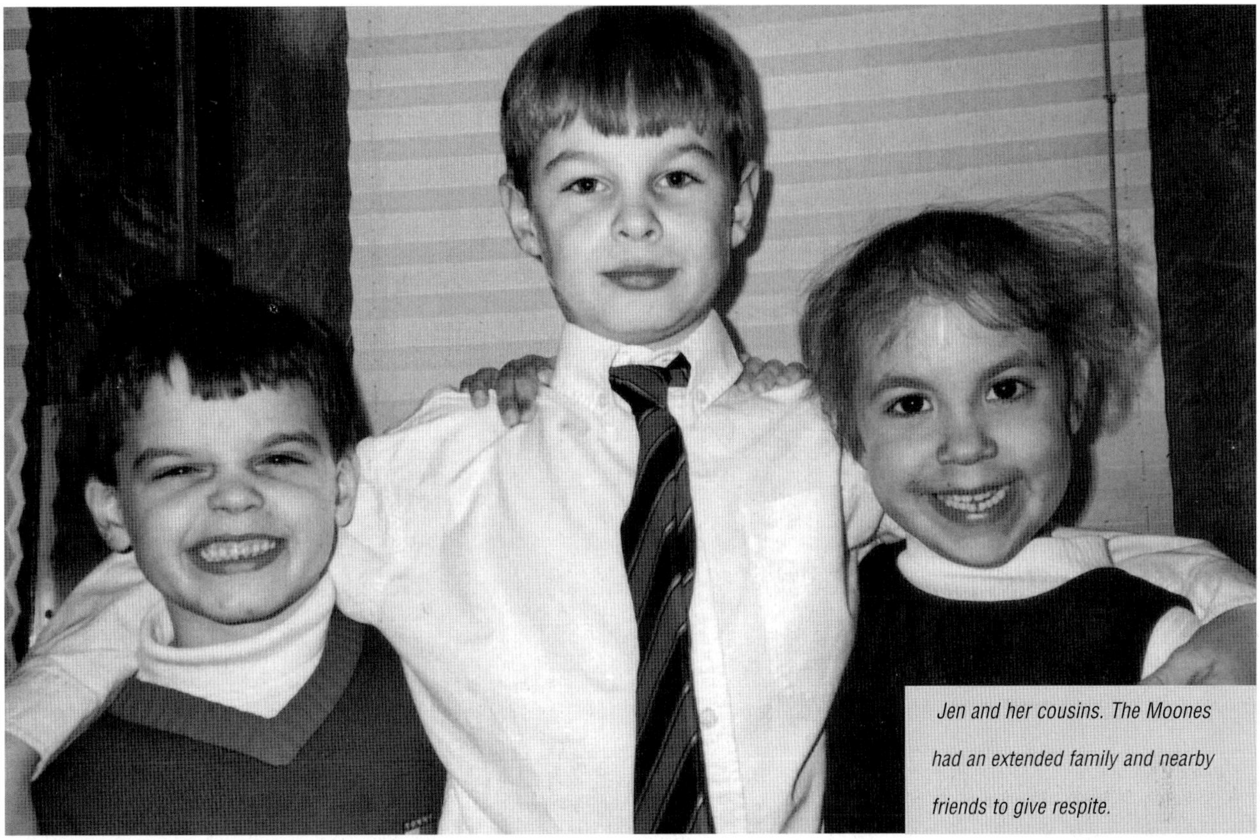

Jen and her cousins. The Moones had an extended family and nearby friends to give respite.

Frank Moone turned down a job transfer to Chicago in 2000 rather than uproot the family and leave the security of living near Cincinnati Children's Hospital.

frankMOONE

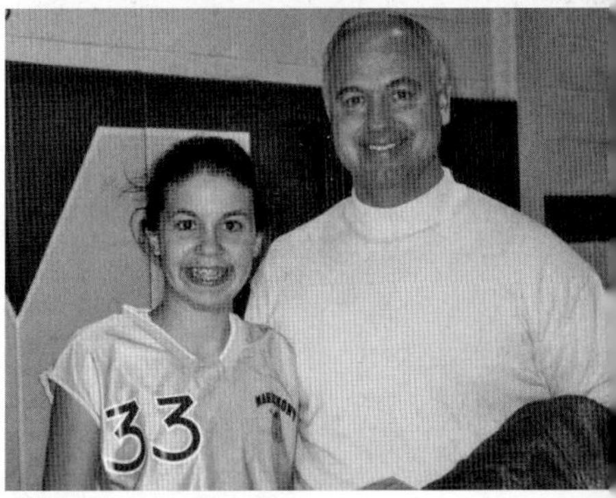

Jen and her sister Natalie are both great, avid basketball players. Dad Frank decided to coach his older daughter's team while Jen was sick, so that Natalie would not be left out.

Just a couple of weeks ago, I was thinking back to the phone call we got. I was sitting on the La-Z-Boy with Jennifer, rocking; Beth got the phone call from the doctor, and I can just remember the trembling in Beth's voice. The look on her face that will stay with me forever and the sinking feeling in your heart, the fear of the unknown. We knew our lives were going to change. I didn't know what leukemia was. I thought it was cancer of the blood, but as far as I was concerned it was terminal. And up to ten years ago, it was.

Every so often you get that reflection back and, gosh, that is what I think about. That little kid is so determined. Whatever she does, she is determined to do well and succeed.

I think if anything I might have withdrawn from co-workers and friends. I am not a real articulate person. If anything, I might have closed up even more. How do you tell somebody your daughter has got cancer? I don't want others' pity or sympathy. Doesn't help anything.

I remember coming home once; they talk about the "moonface," a side effect of the chemotherapy. You come home and it is like you don't even recognize your own child. That was a hard moment. I remember her coming home from the hospital and laying on the couch and just

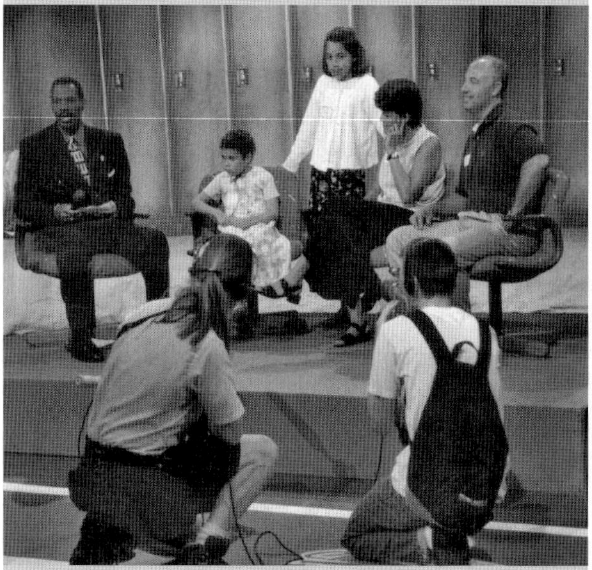

The Moone family was often asked to be interviewed on TV or in newspapers to talk about childhood cancer and raise money for research.

moaning. Those were tough times.

I don't know that I am a very religious person. Spiritual, that's a better word. Personal reflection to God, quiet times; you do a lot of praying.

I think Beth would tell you that you can persevere. You develop a plan, you set your mind to it, you see it through. With God's will, you can persevere. She was very well prepared.

Beth and I kind of took turns being strong. We never fell apart at the same time.

Jennifer Moone remains cancer-free. She plays soccer and basketball and hopes to be a school counselor when she grows up. She attended the Sundance Film Festival for the premiere of A Lion in the House *with her mother.*

I thought the movie was very inspiring, and even though, unfortunately, there are three out of the five families that didn't make it through, there's definitely hope. I'm fourteen years old and I made it through. Al Fields is eighteen and he made it through. So there's definitely good outcomes.

A family friend, Jen, Beth, Natalie and family.

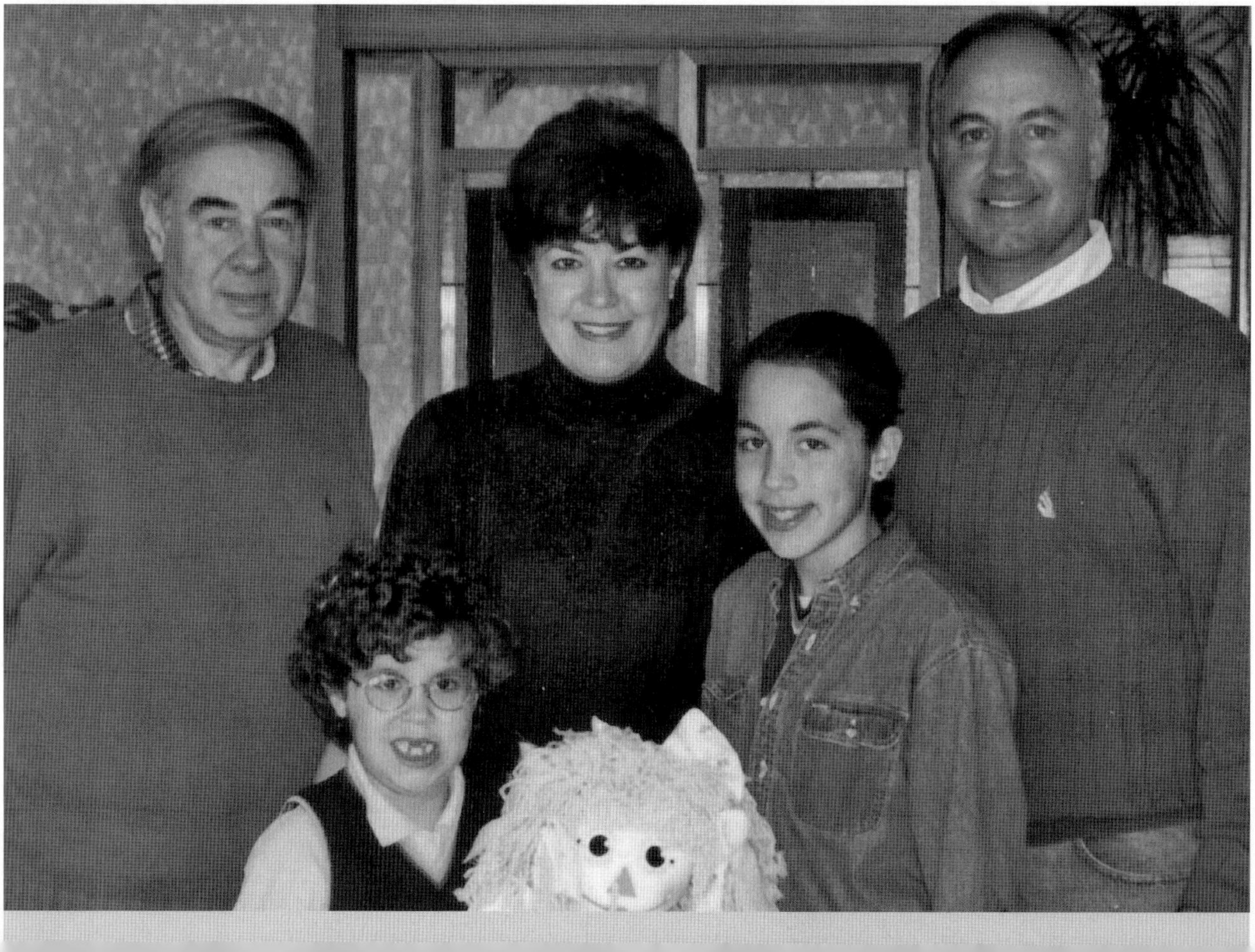

Filmmakers' Journal

Julia: Beth Moone was the person who at first I most identified with, the mom most like me—a college-educated, driven career woman who loved her job, with two beautiful daughters, a great and generous husband, a well organized home life, enjoying all the benefits of the comfortable life they had earned.

It all came to a grinding halt, it all changed on a dime, with the diagnosis. Going through cancer caused her to change her life's priorities. She realized her career orientation and the two-income economic standard was not worth the trade-off of involvement with her daughters' lives.

Beth was raised on a farm, and both her parents were nearby and very able to help. The Moones had close friends nearby who were wonderfully helpful. Her sister was a nurse. It was her urging that alerted Beth to the fact that the pattern of Jen's symptoms might point to leukemia.

Beth and Frank were always gracious, and Beth and I had many long talks, though we honestly never had the opportunity to grow as intimately close to the Moones as to the other families. The Moones and the Fields went through what most families go through with childhood cancer. A terrible shock, a year of hell, maybe more, a reorganization of family life, bumps in the road, then months of their children regaining their footing. Most kids survive cancer! My own daughter almost never had to go to the emergency room or be admitted to the hospital. But that kept us from bonding as closely as we did with the other families, because we didn't go through the very tough times that create those bonds.

Steven: Beth and Frank realized that one of Frank's key roles in all this could really be to support Jen's older sister, Natalie. Like the siblings of Justin, Tim and Alex, Natalie got pushed to the side by the demands of saving her sister's life. It's all very explainable, but still, as Justin's sister Jennifer says, when you're ten or twelve years old, you don't understand. So Frank supported Natalie, particularly by becoming the coach of her basketball team while Jen was still sick. That was a great thing they all shared, and when Natalie became such a basketball whiz, it helped balance out the attention that Jen had been getting. I don't think Jen ever wanted to take attention away from her sister. She never wanted to have the spotlight on her all the time, to the detriment of Natalie.

Julia: Jen was always a well behaved kid, but she also always had this kind of rebel spark, a kind of mischief that hovered right below the surface. I think her doctor, Dr. Cyndi Delaat, brought out the spark in Jen, because Cyndi really appreciates that about kids—their spirit, their humor. So occasionally we'd see moments when Jen would suddenly slap her mom on her butt, stuff like that.

Steven: When Beth ran the (Chicago) marathon, that was really inspiring—that she willed herself, her body, to do that.

Julia: I loved filming her on those early morning summer days. Six a.m. on a country road in southern Ohio in July when the sun is just rising—that was magic.

Steven: Filming the marathon itself was pretty insane. We had no idea what we were getting ourselves into.

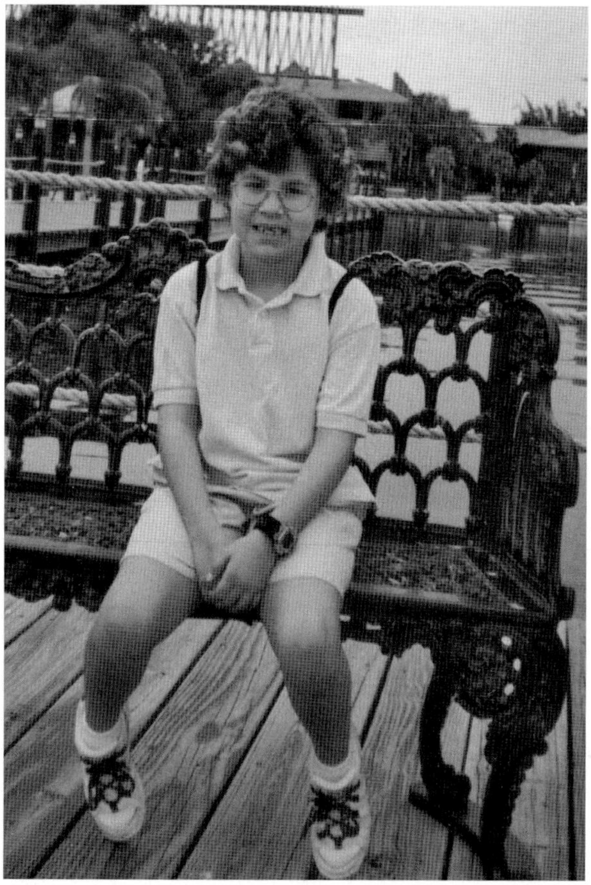

Jen, smiling, though getting sick, at Disneyworld.

Julia: We should have been training ourselves, as much as we walked and ran to shoot it.

Steven: We split into two teams. Julia and a talented young artist, Thea Lux, who had done sound for us several times and who now lived in Chicago, stuck with the Moone family—Frank, Jen, Natalie, Beth's sister, nephews and parents. I went solo, with the job of getting shots of Beth running.

Julia: But we both underestimated how utterly huge this event is. Tens of thousands of runners, over a million people out to watch along the 26 miles of road. How do you find anyone in that kind of crowd?

Steven: I remember getting hypnotized by the sea of faces and color as wave after wave of runners passed by the camera, while I was just hoping against odds that I'd see Beth. I missed her the first few passes. Then I finally found her and got a shot of her passing the camera. After she passed, I realized I'd be an idiot if I didn't get more shots of her right now, while I knew where she was. So I grabbed my heavy backpack and huffed and puffed my way to catch up with her, and then to run ahead of her, and to get another shot. I even did a funny interview with her while we were both running. I did that several times and was completely exhausted before noon.

Julia: It was fun and funny to be hanging out with the Moones in Chicago. Getting donuts, their first time ever riding the subway, surrounded by strange marathon fans. I don't know what we would have done without Thea Lux, because she really knew Chicago, and she kept us from getting lost again and again. By the end of the day, we were all totally exhausted. It took a week for our bodies to recover.

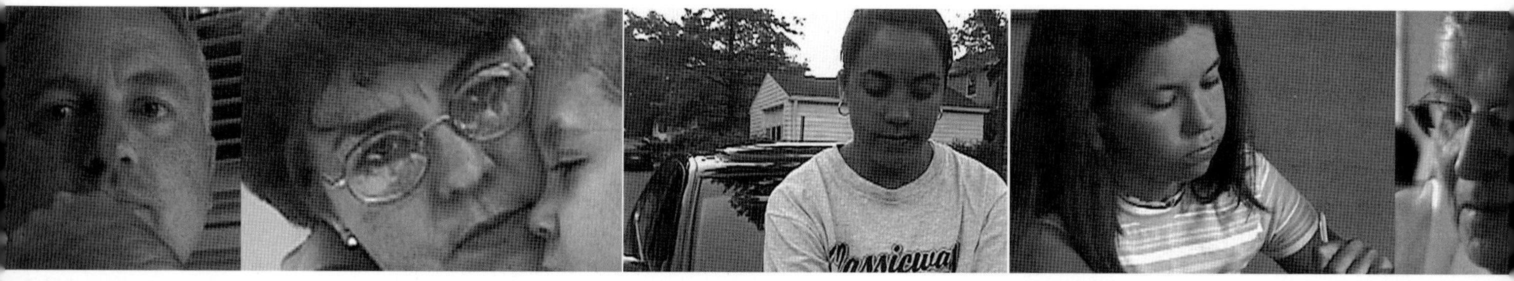

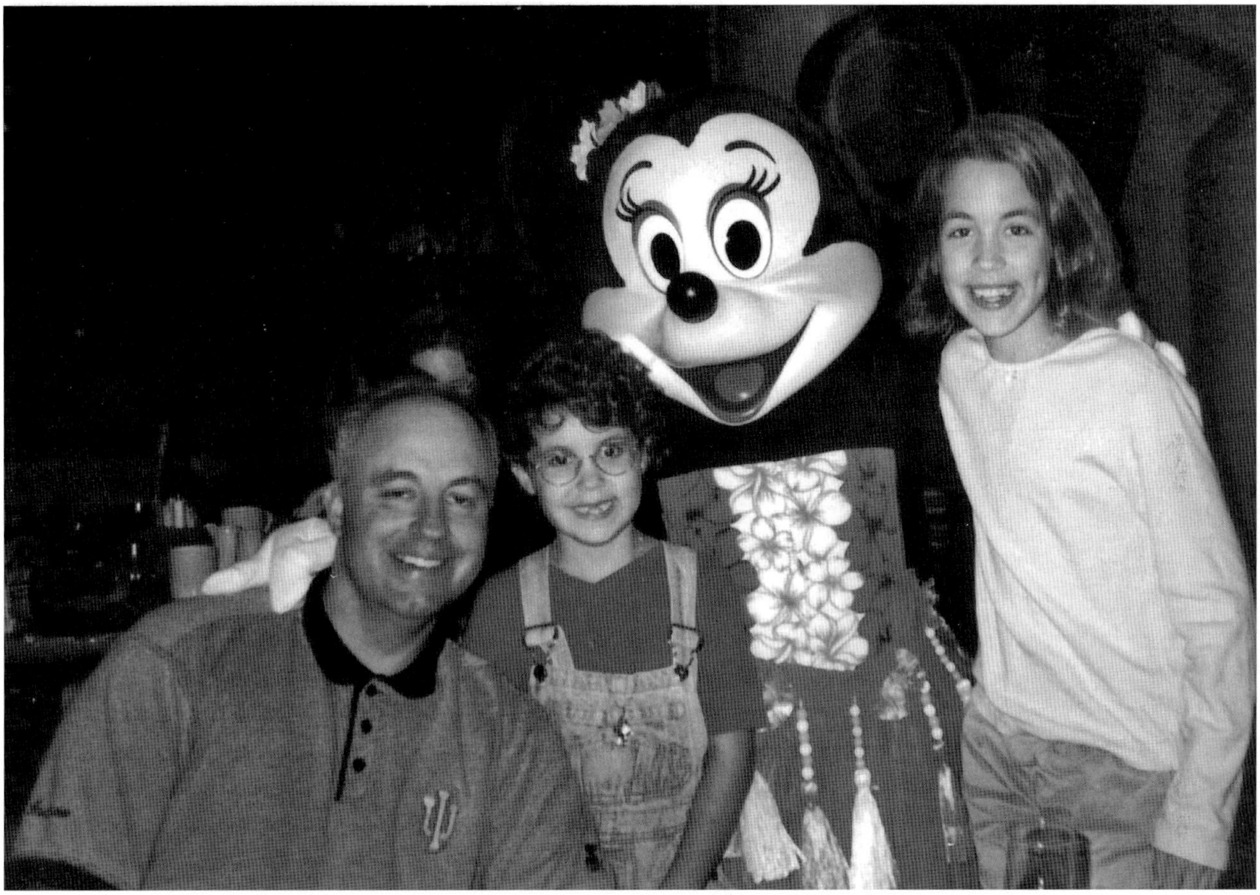

Jen and her family got a Special Wish trip to Disneyworld. The whole family got a touch of food poisoning while there, but Jen became extremely sick and was hospitalized for two weeks.

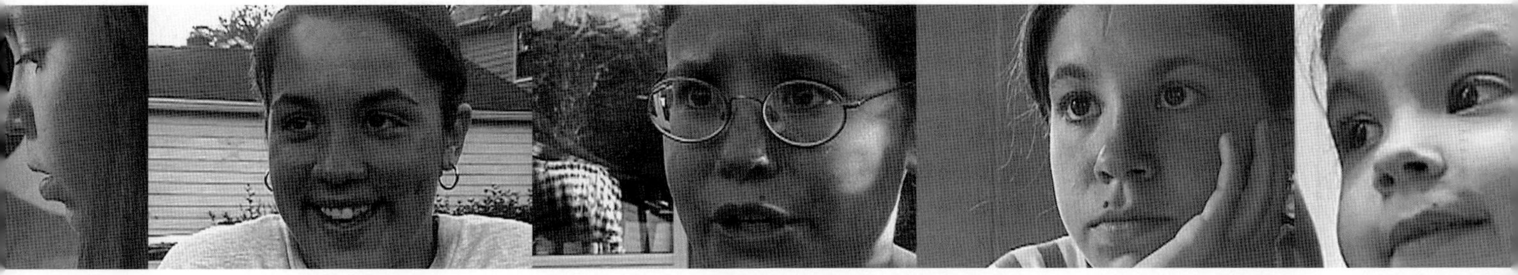

Chapter 3

Timothy WOODS

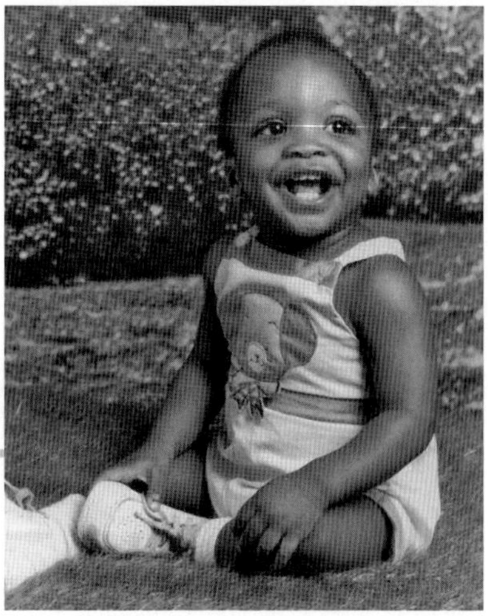

Tim was Marietha's firstborn child.

mariethaWOODS

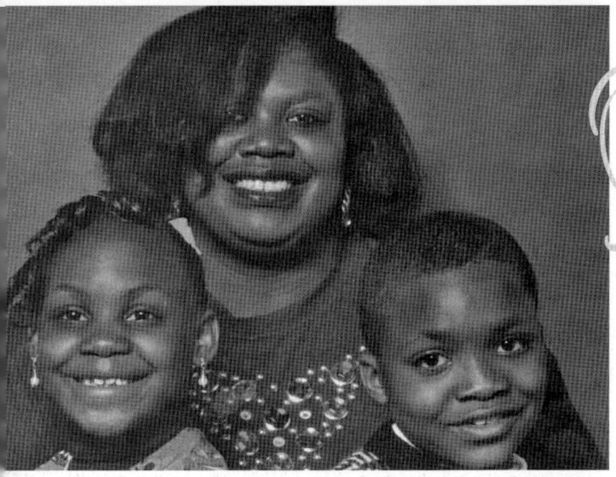

Marietha Woods with her two children, Taletha and Tim.

Tim's mother raised him and his younger sister Taletha on her own. Tim's father was murdered in 1995. Marietha also took care of several relatives who shared her home, including her infant nephew Tyrik, whom Marietha unofficially adopted before Tim became ill and whom everyone regarded as Tim's little brother.

When Tim was a baby, he was a very picky eater. Hyper, hyper, hyper, hyper and a crybaby. He had big ole crocodile tears. He was a mama's and grandma's baby. He had to be up on either one of us.

He was always busy somewhere doing something. He wasn't always doing anything bad or anything. He loved to collect rocks. He was always going into other people's gardens and picking flowers. He was a good kid. If he got a little money taking out somebody's garbage or whatever, he always found a way to buy me something. He was a sweet kid. He was silly, bubbly, fun to be around.

When I first got Tyrik, I stopped working (at a local bank). I didn't trust anyone to watch him, so I had done all my paperwork to be a daycare provider and get certified and everything. Then Tim got sick. I got Tyrik in January, and Tim got sick that June.

When I was working, I still had paychecks coming in, and we still did family things, family weekends. Then after he got sick, people started moving in, and it just spiraled down from there.

I thought it was asthma. So I took him to a clinic, and they told me he had strep throat and a chest cold. That Monday he was supposed to go to camp. We both overslept, which I think is the grace of God, because I took him to St. Francis/St. George (Hospital) and they sent me over here. They said if he went to camp, he would have died because the tumor was so big it was collapsing his windpipe. They said he wouldn't have made it through the whole week at camp.

They said it looks like Hodgkins lymphoma. I said, "What in the world is that?" They said "It's a rare form of cancer, but not as rare as it used to be. It's highly treatable and curable." I said, "Okay, it's curable." But he was so sick they couldn't even do a CT scan.

I don't remember him crying. I just remember him being spacey looking and saying, "Well, Mom, we'll beat it."

He was in the hospital more than he was out, honestly, except for that little time he went in the summer between July to September (1998). In October, they started seeing signs. It got progressively bad. In November, we went to Chicago (on a vacation arranged by hospital personnel and funded by McDonald's, where Tim worked). December, January—then he was gone. He did a lot of his time on the inside.

When you are in a situation like that, you cannot be anything but honest. You cannot sugarcoat anything. You cannot lie about nothing. It's bold and real. If your child has cancer you can't just say, "Oh, he's just got a cold." You cannot take that lightly. To take it seriously, you have to be truthful.

At the time of diagnosis, Tim was 14. Coping with the disease was a reality. He knew he had this disease, but at the same time he wanted to be a kid. To be a kid means he couldn't walk around taking medicine three to five times a day. It limited him in a lot of things that he couldn't do. I think he thought if I'm going to be rebellious, I'm going to be rebellious all the way. I'm not going to take the medicine. I'm not going to do what they tell me. I'm just going to do what I'm going to do because I'm a kid—till I get busted.

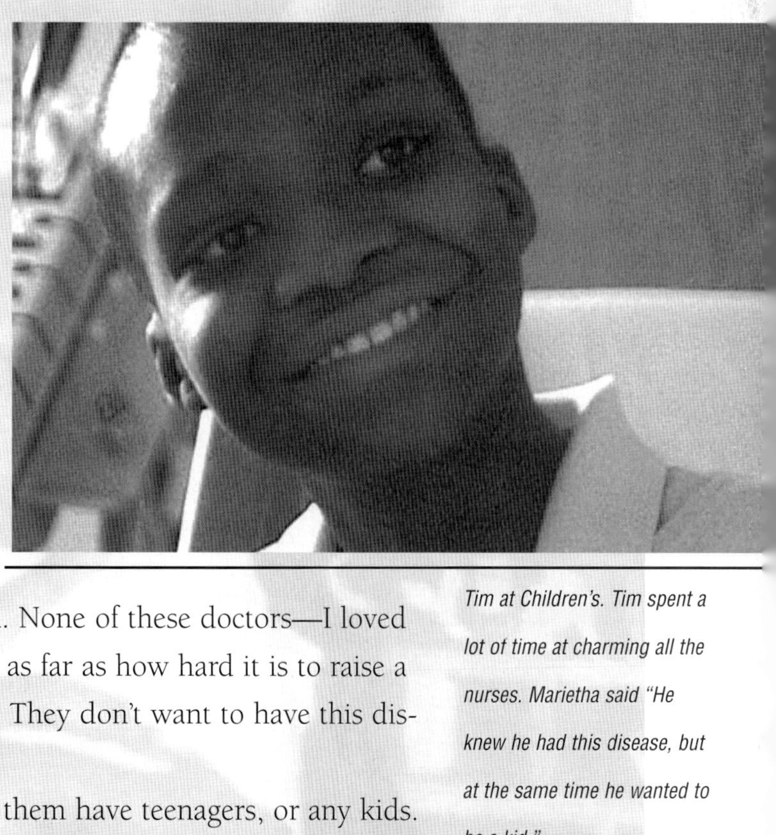

Tim at Children's. Tim spent a lot of time at charming all the nurses. Marietha said "He knew he had this disease, but at the same time he wanted to be a kid."

The doctors, they were nice. Dr. Arceci, he was the best. I don't have one bad thing to say about him. None of these doctors—I loved them all, but some of them weren't as understanding as far as how hard it is to raise a teenager and be a single parent and he was rebelling. They don't want to have this disease. They don't want to be sick.

Some of the nurses understood, because some of them have teenagers, or any kids. I couldn't be in his presence 24-7. They were saying, "You are the mother. You should be doing this." Well, those were the people who didn't have kids. The ones who had kids, they understood. If you want to live in my house and be with a sick child 24

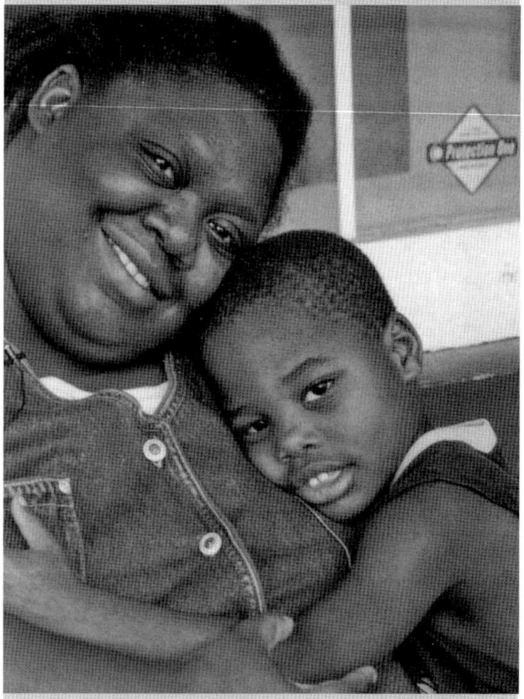

Marietha & Tyrik on her front porch. Marietha adopted Tyrik, her brother's baby son, to keep him from going in the foster care system. Though Tyrik eventually moved back in with his birth mother, he remains close to Marietha.

hours a day, then you will see. Until then, don't judge me, because you don't know what I go through every day. You don't know that I don't have a big support group. I have a lot of family members, but just because I have a lot of family members, doesn't mean they are supporting me through this. You can have seven sisters and out of seven, maybe one will help you.

I had family members right in my household, but when it came time to take Tyrik to his checkup, I couldn't get one of them to take him.

If I had to take the baby to the doctor, I had to wait till Tim was on the blood transfusion machine, get up and run the baby across the street to the clinic. I wasn't supposed to leave him because he was getting a blood transfusion, so what was I supposed to do? It was hard trying to take care of this baby and try to take care of him.

Taletha needed things done. It got to the point that I wasn't spending enough time with her and she started rebelling. It seemed like I loved him more than her, and it wasn't that. I was spread too thin.

Me being as physically tired as I was, was no good for him. When I ended up sick I had laryngitis, the flu and a touch of pneumonia at the same time. If he had caught any of those germs it would have been ten times worse for him. So, I couldn't go to the hospital because I was sick. Nobody else was home. They'd call me on the phone and say, "Oh, no, don't come." But after three or four days they expected me to jump up as super mom and be over there again. Then it got to the stage that I wasn't coming and "I was neglecting." It was like you couldn't win in certain situations. No matter what I did, somebody was hurt.

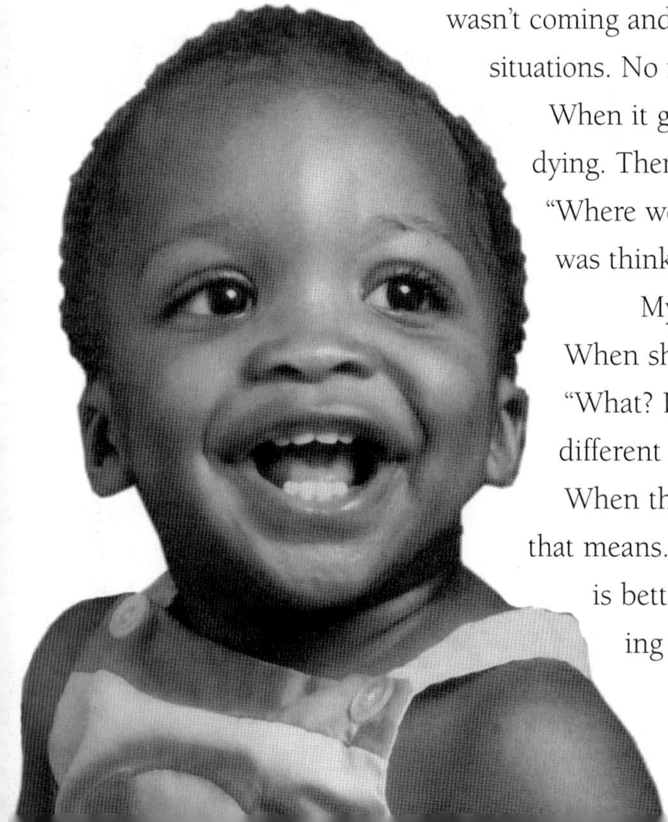

When it got down to the wire and they saw how serious it was, he was dying. Then you couldn't get people away from the hospital. I thought, "Where were you at all these other times?" That's what I dealt with. I was thinking, "It's the end now. I needed you then!"

My mother died of cancer (at age fifty), but she never told us. When she died, the doctor said, "Well, the cancer. . ." I was like, "What? I thought she had heart trouble!" I wish I knew more about different forms of cancer and how they are treated.

When they give you odds, I would have liked to have known what that means. "Well, he has an 80 percent cure rate." Okay, I assume that is better than 50 percent, but at the same time when you are dealing with cancer, that can be nothing. It's the luck of the draw.

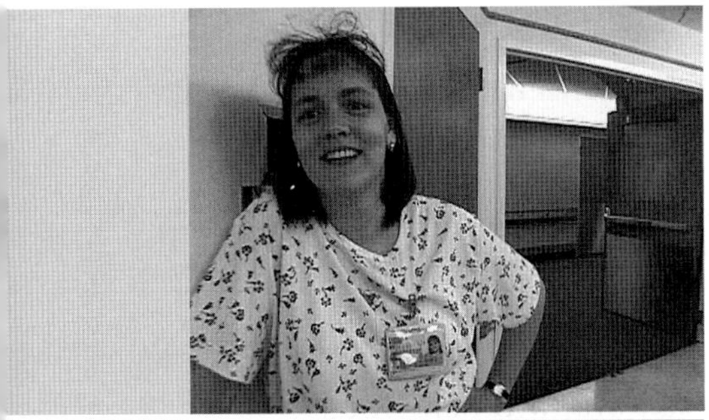

Tim's nurse Connie Koons.

Not that I felt I would have needed a second opinion, but I wish I had another doctor that I could ask, "Is this the best course of treatment? Is there something else out there?"

Tim was like the hospital's child. All the nurses wanted to take him home. All the doctors wanted to take him home. He even went to Steve and Julia's house overnight one time. He's been everywhere. Connie and Rob (Tim's favorite nurse and her husband) took him home a lot. Especially when he was really well and could go places.

He was protective of Taletha, but at the same time she was protective of him. Like if any girls ever hit Tim, she'd bust them up. The same thing went with Taletha; if any boys walloped her, he'd bust them up. They fought like cats and dogs. You had the sibling rivalry, and then the "I love you so much." This is the same thing my brothers and sisters went through. You'd wring their neck one minute and beat the world up for them the next.

I don't think Tim stopped liking school till he lost all that weight. His friends wouldn't hang around with him. They wanted to know what was wrong with him. "Oh, you've got a disease. We don't want to catch it!"

Tim was a sleeper. I would roam the halls while he was sleeping. I would just roam the halls and play with the babies at the window. There wasn't a whole lot to do up there for adults. That's another thing they could change. I know it's a children's hospital and it's equipped for the kids, but they need more things for adults to do. If they want us there 24-7, make it more comfortable for us too. They could have a room where adults can go to play board games. They have that big old room where kids can go to play games or Playstations. Adults need a stress release too. They need to set-up a room for us: maybe a big screen TV or a room to play music or something to kick back and unwind.

Six-year-old Tim Woods in his kindergarten class. Tim enjoyed school until he got sick at fourteen. After that, he missed a great deal of school, fell farther and farther behind, and disliked going.

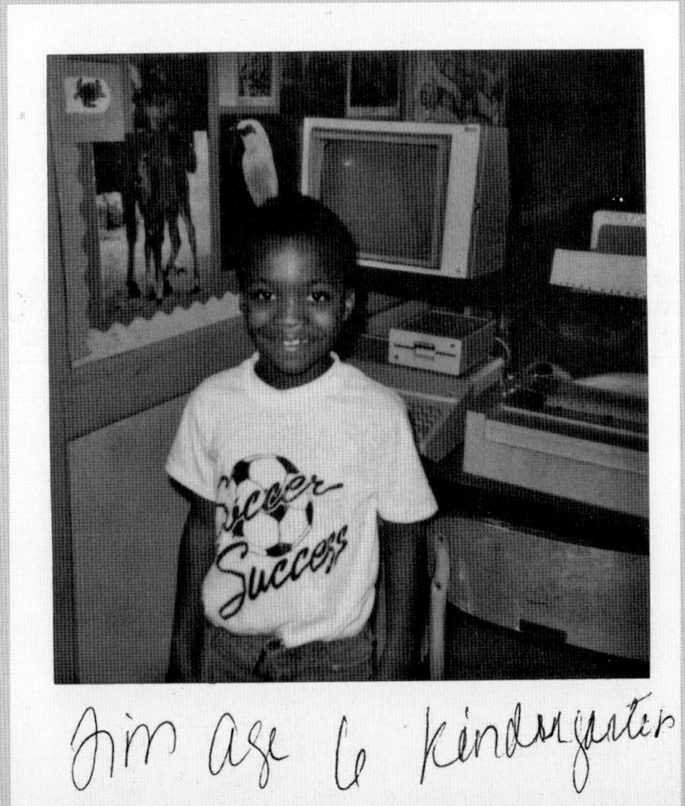

I'm talking about us that's up on the floors when we have been there for days and weeks at a time. We were doing our laundry there. That's how long I was there. He was in the ICU for like 15 days and I did not leave for one day. I about lost my mind because I didn't have nothing to do. I love to clean. Every time they came in to clean his room, they didn't have anything to clean. I cleaned everything.

My son's social worker—she was a sweet lady, don't get me wrong—my son called me one day and he was hysterically crying. She had been in there with this other guy and they discussed Hospice with him. I wasn't there. That terrified him because of the way she was coming at him: "You are going to die."

That's not the way you should go to a child, just bluntly like that. I was really pissed. Nobody had a clue why she went in that room and told him that. None of his doctors told her to do it. You did not have the right to do that, nor did you have the parent's permission to do that. It took four days to get him right in the head. He was hysterical and literally sick from fear. I did not know he was dying. That pissed me off cause nobody came and told me, "We are not doing anything else. There's nothing else we can do."

As Tim's cancer grew worse, his doctors offered him a last-ditch choice between two intensive chemotherapies.

He was so tired of taking drugs towards the end, so I just kind of left that decision up to him. The only problem I had was, "If it's not really going to help him, then what is the use?"

I wanted something that was going to help him where eventually he could be not doing this anymore—cured, basically.

What they were telling me, we could give him this chemo or we could give him that chemo. It seemed like the luck of the draw. It got to be too experimental for me. Outside of that, they were always clear with me. It wasn't like they were leaving out tidbits of information. When it got to the experimental stages, they were just trying stuff to see maybe if it would catch on and work. It got too much for him because he had gotten so small, he had to wear the brace. The chemo started eating away his tissue and he was just skin and bone, and weak. This was getting to be too much.

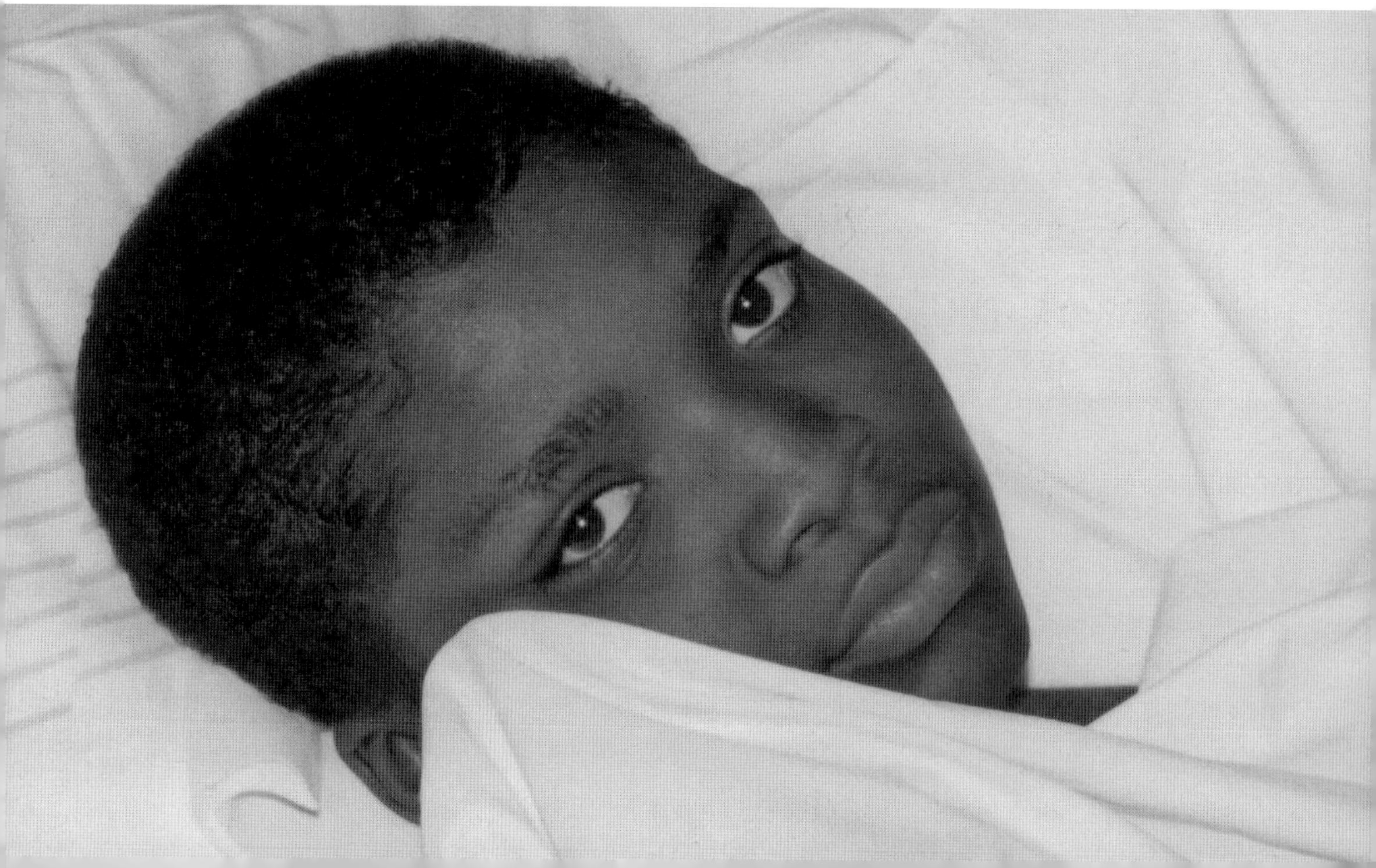

You don't want to think about giving up on your child. At the same time you can look at your child and tell they can't take no more. You don't want your child to be on this earth just because you don't want to lose him. As opposed to, he's on this earth, but he's suffering so bad. You are supposed to love him. Why would you want him to be in that kind of pain?

When you get to that point where enough is enough, you've really weighed all the options. If I do this, will it make him better? Looking at him now, he's wasting away. Is this better for him? Will it make a difference?

Then I had to ask him. He wasn't no little bitty kid. He was sixteen. I asked him, "Tim, if you want to fight, I will fight with you. If you are tired, you are tired. I can't make you feel like you have to do something because of me. It's not about me, it's about you." He just said he wanted to fight. That's when we decided to do the chemo. His body couldn't take it. I knew that, but it was his decision about *his* body.

You got one child you want to make well and one you try to shelter. She wanted to be up there to see him *(Taletha, who was eleven at the time, regrets not seeing Tim in his last days)*. But he's either running a fever from the chemo, he's got sores in his mouth, he doesn't eat. When he does eat, he throws it up. I thought that she at that age did not need to see that. That would have made it worse for her. She was already rebelling. I think that would have pushed her over a little bit more.

As Tim neared death, Marietha wanted to take him home, but he stayed in the hospital. I didn't decide not to; *he* decided not to. I asked him how he felt about going home. He said, "No. I think I'll stay here a few more days till I feel a little better." I said, "The doctor said I could take you home." He said, "No, I'd rather wait until I feel a little better." I said, "Well, okay." I figured whatever happens, happens. I couldn't tell him, "Tim you are going to die in a week. Do you want to go home?" If he did have any determination to fight, that would have killed him.

The next day, I could tell that his breathing was different. He was still walking and could talk. When I went up there that Friday, he was pretty much in a coma. He died early that Saturday morning. He wouldn't have been home a day before he died.

They were telling me after that it was just as well he didn't go home. If I had fallen asleep and woke up with him lying there dead or something like that, I probably would have freaked out. I was just thinking, "If he's going to die, I want him around home with me. I didn't want him in this hospital around strangers." But thank God we were all there when it happened.

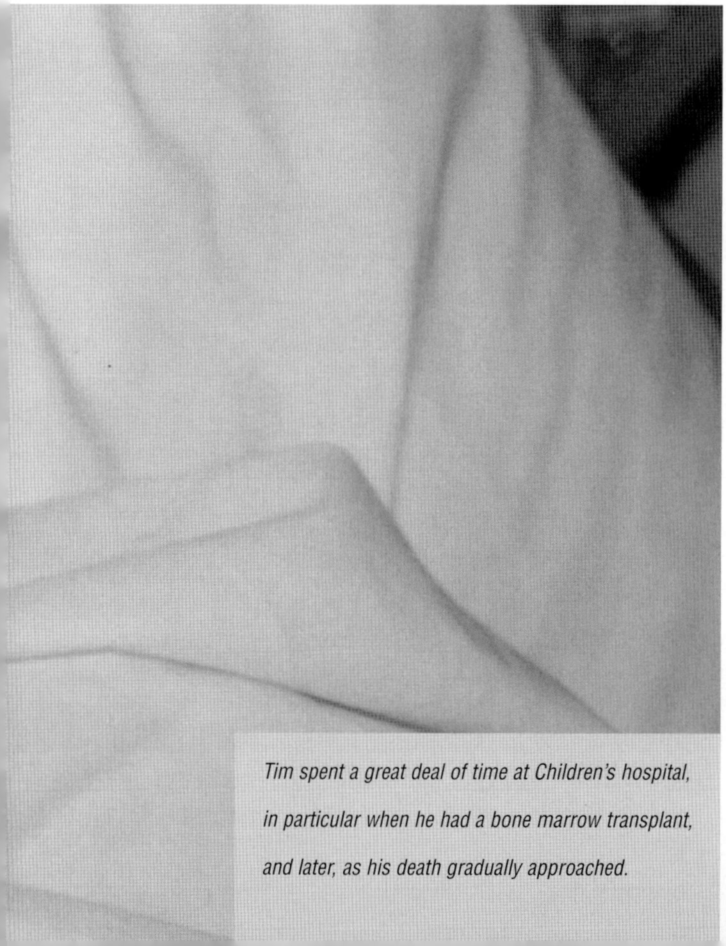

Tim spent a great deal of time at Children's hospital, in particular when he had a bone marrow transplant, and later, as his death gradually approached.

After Tim died, I started going to counseling. The first thing they wanted to do is put me on drugs. I had to work to get government assistance. The only reason I wasn't working was because he got sick. I told him I was trying to find a job. He said, "Until you find a job, we are going to put you in a support group." I was like, fine, but they wanted to put me in a support group with crack heads. I didn't want to be with no crack heads. I was dealing with grief.

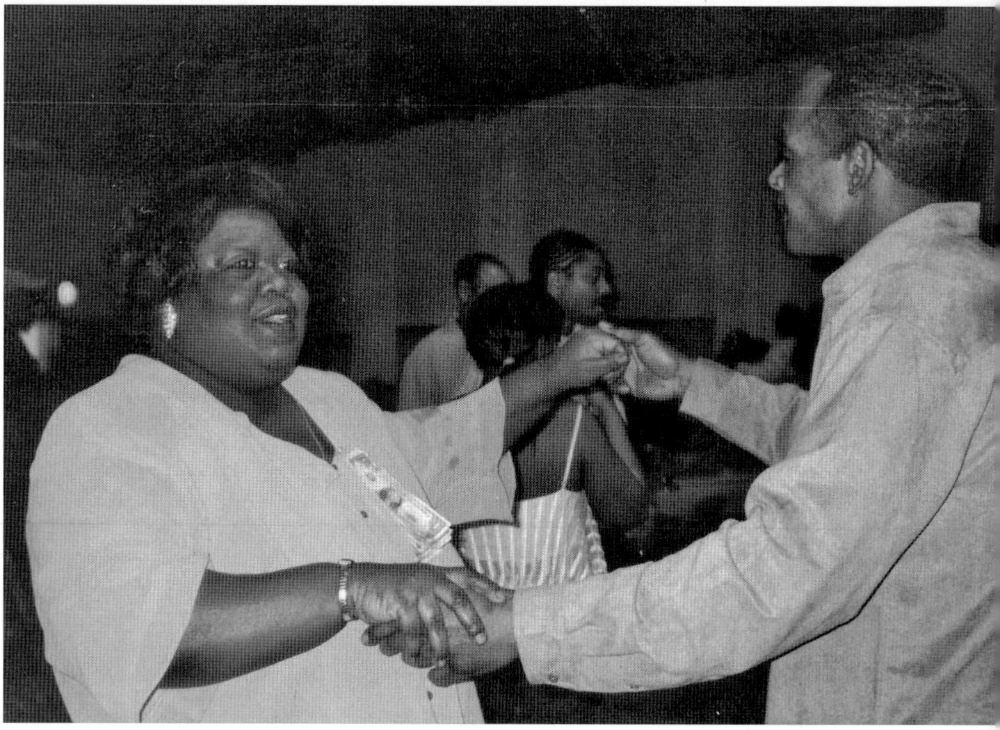

Marietha Woods dances with her fiancé, Ron Thomas, at her 40th birthday party in 2005.

I ended up getting into this, what is it called, where you go to an individual psychiatrist. As soon as I got there, this lovely lady pulls out this pad and she starts writing down my information. I'm looking and there's a prescription pad. She was writing out Xanax, Prozac. She didn't even ask about me and why am I depressed.

I'm like, "Why are you writing out these prescriptions?" She said, "Well, you know you are depressed, and these can help you function." I was like, I can function fine. I wasn't so much depressed as sad. She said, "These will help you feel better."

Needless to say I didn't fill the prescriptions. They sat on my desk and collected dust. I didn't go back. That was not for me. At least she could have heard what I'm going through. If she had listened two or three sessions, I would have felt better taking the prescriptions. I got away from that. I pretty much winged it and got around some family and friends. I was okay after that.

There's been times when I've been sitting in the house and I'll think I hear him talking. Or a cool breeze will go across my back. Or like echoes. Just weird things. I can hear somebody walking around upstairs. I thought I would be scared or something like that, but I just hear and go "Ah," and go on about my business. Tyrik would be sitting there talking, and I'm like, "Tyrik, who are you talking to?" "Tim." And you know, I'm like, "Okay," and I leave him alone, 'cause maybe he is. I don't know.

Being born is a blessing no matter what color you are. Being able to live to the age that I am in this world is another blessing. You've got kids shooting each other in schools. That stuff didn't happen when I was coming up. You've got drive-bys. You could leave your doors unlocked when I was coming up. You can't now. So a whole lot of things I'm blessed with no matter what color I am.

If I feel like someone is being racist to me, I deal with them right there directly to their face. I make them accept what they've done, what they've said to me, and make them know that they were out of order. You're not going to get away with that with me. So I don't have a problem with racism, not at all.

Life is precious and too short and it's here and gone in the blink of an eye. And how you choose to live it in your blink is up to you. I choose not to live my life on (racial) terms and dwell on that. I don't have a problem with racism. I have a problem with relationships (laughs).

Anybody who's been around me all my years of life could tell you that the one main thing for sure is that I've always taken care of my children, no matter what I've done, when I've done it. I've always taken care of my children, always made sure they were fed, dry, they had clean clothes, new clothes.

He would be twenty-two going on twenty-three now. He was such a comedian. He was really funny. He always said he wanted to be a doctor/lawyer/football player. I would say, "You are going to spread yourself pretty thin."

He'd say, "Well, you can have the car and house that you need and deserve. I need the car and house I need and deserve. We'll have Taletha to be the babysitter." That was his sister's job. Come to find out that she doesn't have a lick of patience with kids. If he was living now, I don't know if he would have kids now or not. He would be graduated and might have been going to college or something. He would basically be the comedian and nut that he was.

talethaWOODS

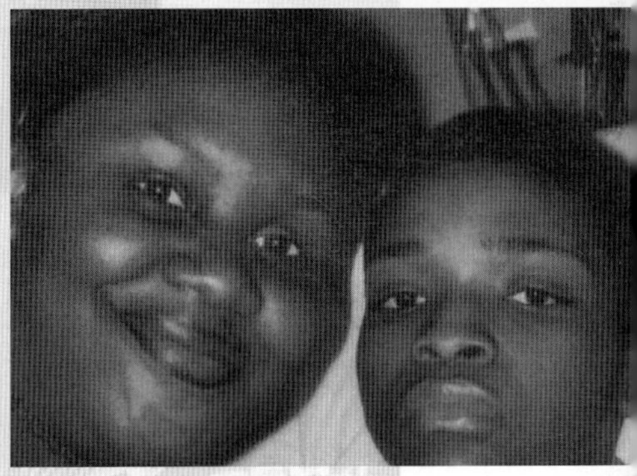

Taletha and Tim "chillin' on New Year's Eve."

Tim's younger sister, Taletha Woods, is now the mother of a toddler; she lives with Marietha in northern Ohio.

It was hard, yeah, real hard for me. My mom left me with aunts and I was stuck doing housework. I felt like I was in prison. I couldn't go outside. I had to clean up their messes. I had to sit inside the whole day till my mom came home.

I was just miserable without my mom—and my brother, 'cause I didn't have nobody to argue with and tell me that I look cute. I didn't have anyone to tell me to, "Be in the house by this time." You know—big brother!

Sometimes we'd get on each other's nerves, but we loved each other. We understood each other. That was the good thing about it. When he left, I just felt all by myself. Like the song says: No more arguing, no more telling me how I look, no more teaching me math. He got straight A's. Yeah, that's how I learned multiplication. He sat at the table and taught me. He was kind of nerdy and loved school. I was slower at learning than he was. It was getting hard for me. I'd hear words from other people about how slow I am and how slow I'm doing in school. My grades dropped from D's to F's.

After he passed, my mom was around more, but I didn't want to talk to her. I didn't know how to talk to her to be honest. I just shut down. I didn't want to go nowhere for that first week. I didn't want to talk to anybody.

My family wasn't there either. My aunts and my uncles, they were there physically, but not in an emotional sense. They were there because they had to be there. They weren't there to talk to me or tell me it was going to be okay or hug me. Nothing.

I had the Salvation Army. I used to go to church there. It wasn't family, it wasn't friends, but at least somebody cared. At the time when it was all going on I resented (my relatives). They were supposed to be my family. They had their own kids. They weren't happy about watching me. That's when I felt I had to start acting up to get attention. That didn't work.

I actually cut myself. I never told my mom that. I have little scars. I felt like that pain would be so much easier than the inside pain I was feeling now. It would have been easier to bleed.

Trying to cut yourself is basically trying to kill yourself and give up on somebody who needs you. My brother needed me and I didn't want to give up. I let him know that I was here. I tried again after he died. I didn't think I could live without my brother.

Then I thought about my mom. She would have two kids gone. She would flip, so I stopped again. After he died, yeah, I was doing that and I was smoking, drinking and hanging out with the wrong people. I went to jail twice.

That wasn't me. I was putting my mom through pain. She had just gone through pain. To see that it wasn't worth it basically. I stopped hanging out with the mean crowd and got my stuff together.

We went to counseling. It helped a lot. I didn't participate at first. I just sat there. I got used to it, though. They had little cards if you didn't want to talk and you had a question, they would talk to you privately. The first week I did that. After that I started being sociable with everybody. It really did help. I got my grades back up. I started getting honor rolls and certificates. I graduated with a 4.0. I was happy.

The Woods family enjoyed Chicago: the Navy Pier, the Aquarium, window shopping on the Miracle Mile, and the beautiful lakefront.

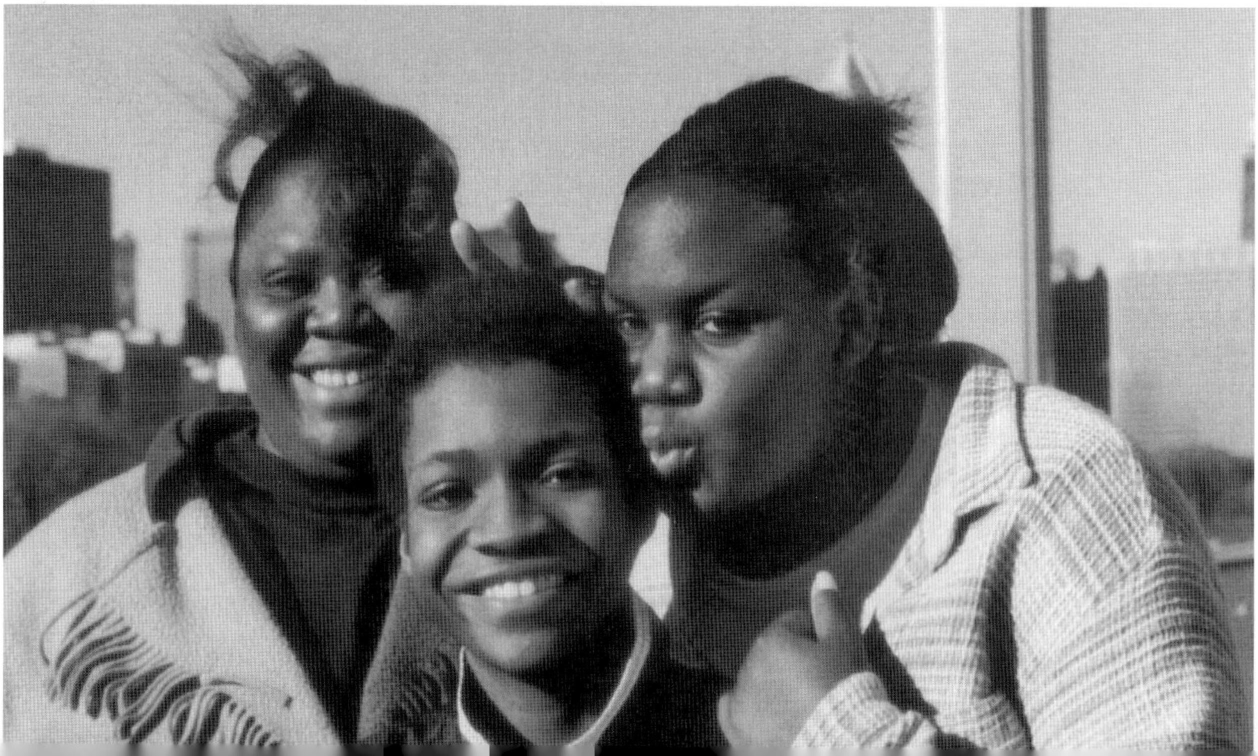

Filmmakers' Journal

Julia: We met Marietha and Tim and Taletha and I think Tyrik at the hospital's annual picnic for their families. Marietha was very warm and accepting. She liked us, it seemed, right away, and there were no barriers. She was funny and ribald. Wickedly funny.

The day we met them, we drove their extended family home, in two cars. For some reason, Steve and I had each driven down that day. And they were all making fun of what a slow driver Steve was. They'd just met us and there were immediately no pretensions.

They were always living on the edge, it seemed, financially, but people still flocked to her house, Marietha was still the matriarch, and many people came to her for advice. She was a homebody, did not like to travel.

Steven: Marietha has had such a life, and I wish this was in the film in some way. She has been through so much, and has walked so many different roads. She described herself to us in one of the interviews as a street person. I asked her what did that mean. She said something like, "A street person is a person who knows how to survive, how to get by, how to make it." The stories she told of herself as a young woman running around, they were really scary and funny all at once. One aspect of that is that when she was a teenager, she looked like she was in her twenties. She talked about hanging out with women in their twenties when she was, like, fifteen, and how they introduced her to stuff—not all good stuff—and how that shaped her.

Julia: I just think of Tim as extremely engaging. He was almost like a stand-up comedian. Adorable, with that thousand-watt smile. The thing about Tim is he was always so quicksilver. He always had stuff to say, and he was so fast at conversation. But he could grow moody, as if a cloud was going by, and he would get quiet. There were just a few times when he would talk about that. One of them is in the film, when he talks to Steve about why he drinks.

Connie described meeting Tim, and her first impression, that he was a chunky kid with a mouth on him and he was just a hoot. I could see that. But through his relapse and bone marrow transplant and periods of solitude, he always maintained an air of dignity and hope.

Steven: Tim had the ability to find joy in life. Regardless of the situation, he had a kind of divining rod to find a laugh or a spark in any situation.

Julia: Tim was so observant, he caught everything. Very interested in people, unusual for a teenager. Oh, he

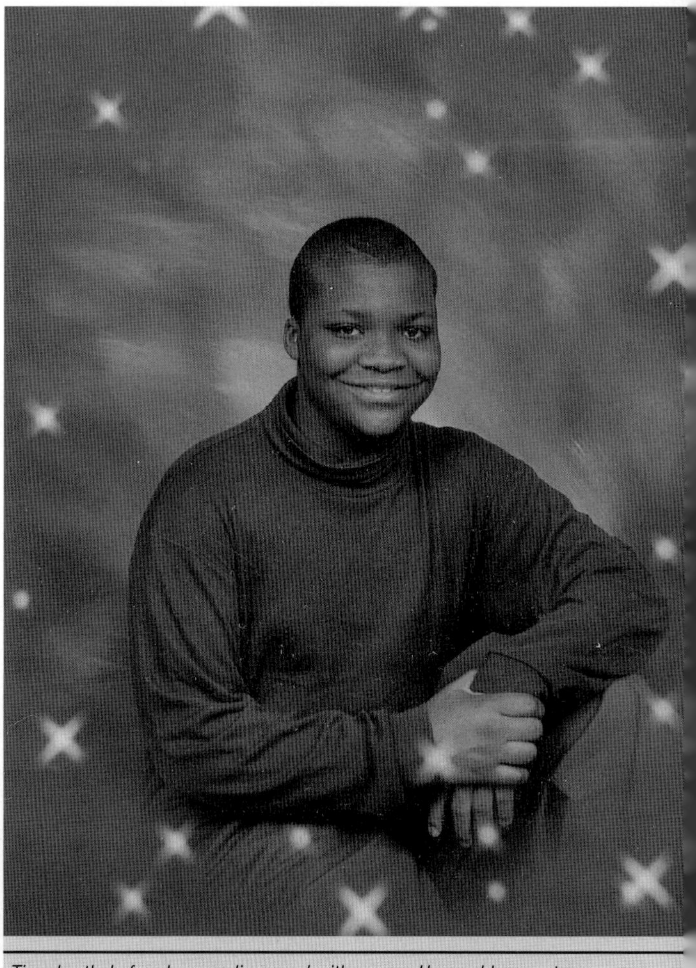

Tim shortly before he was diagnosed with cancer. He would go on to lose a lot of weight after treatments began.

would have the ability to poke endless fun at people. But kind, too; he'd never fully cross the line. He wasn't ever mean.

Tim had huge dreams, and he talked about them often, dreams of buying a farm for his mom and sister, of having a big salt water fish tank, of being a doctor, of going to college, of travel. He really wanted to travel, to see the world. Steve and I traveled quite a bit during the years we knew Tim, and he always wanted to know about the place, the people.

Steven: Tim's little brother Tyrik was a total thief of hearts. That little boy would charm everyone he met, even at Children's Hospital, where there's no shortage of adorable kids. But he was a dynamo too. It was all Marietha and Tim and sometimes Julia and I could do to keep him from making trouble. One time, when we were all standing in a waiting room, he ran off toward the elevator bank. None of us moved fast enough, and before we know it, this two-year-old has dashed into an empty elevator, and is reaching up for the buttons. The elevator door closes. We all look at each other and realize—he could be going *anywhere* in the hospital. It was really scary and really funny all at once. The elevator eventually came back and thank goodness he was still on it.

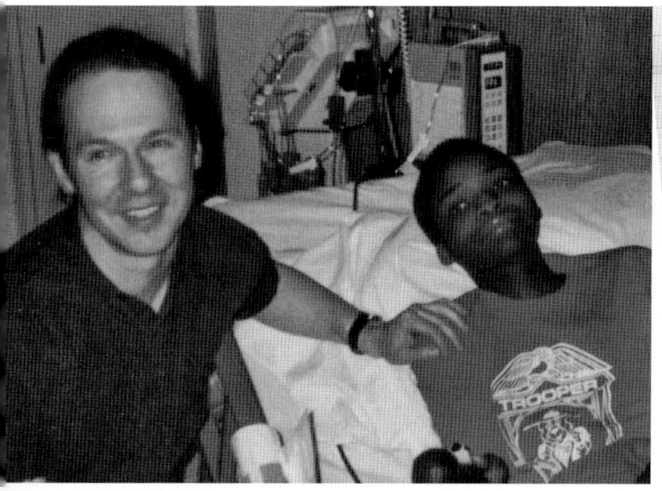

Tim and filmmaker Steven Bognar hanging out at Children's on New Year's Eve.

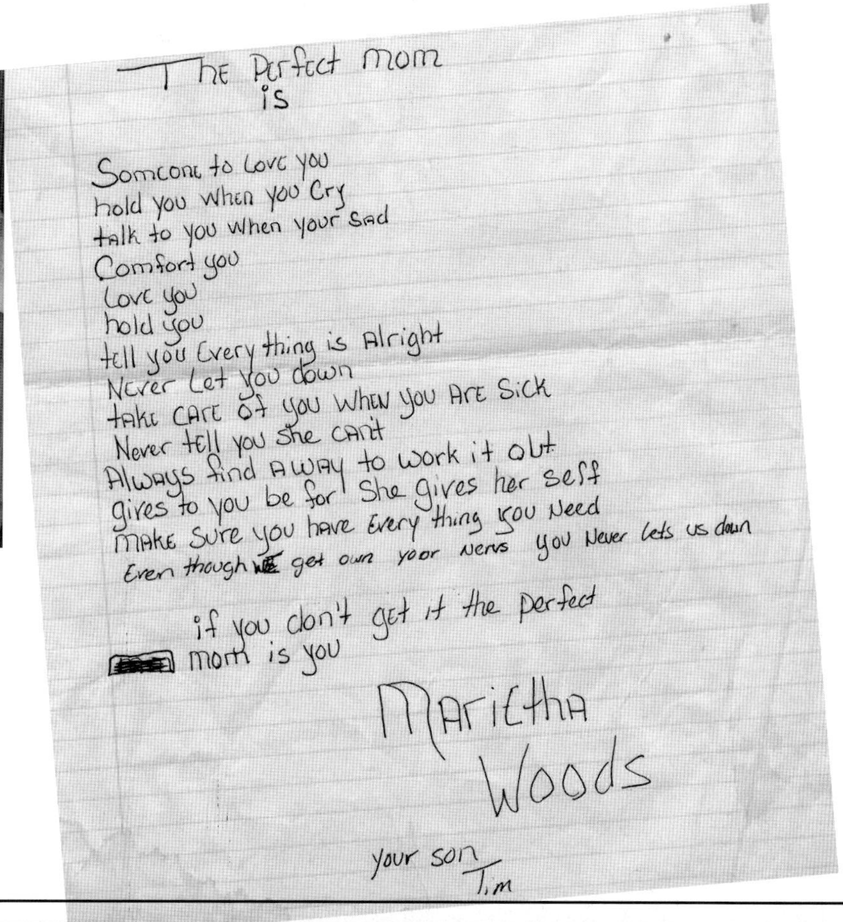

The Perfect mom
is

Somcone to Love you
hold you when you Cry
talk to you when your Sad
Comfort you
Love you
hold you
tell you Every thing is Alright
Never Let you down
take CAre of you when you Are Sick
Never tell you she CAn't
Always find A wAy to work it out
gives to you be for She gives her seff
mAke Sure you have Every thing you Need
Even though we get own yoor nervs you Never lets us down

if you don't get it the perfect
mom is you

MAriEthA
Woods

your son
Tim

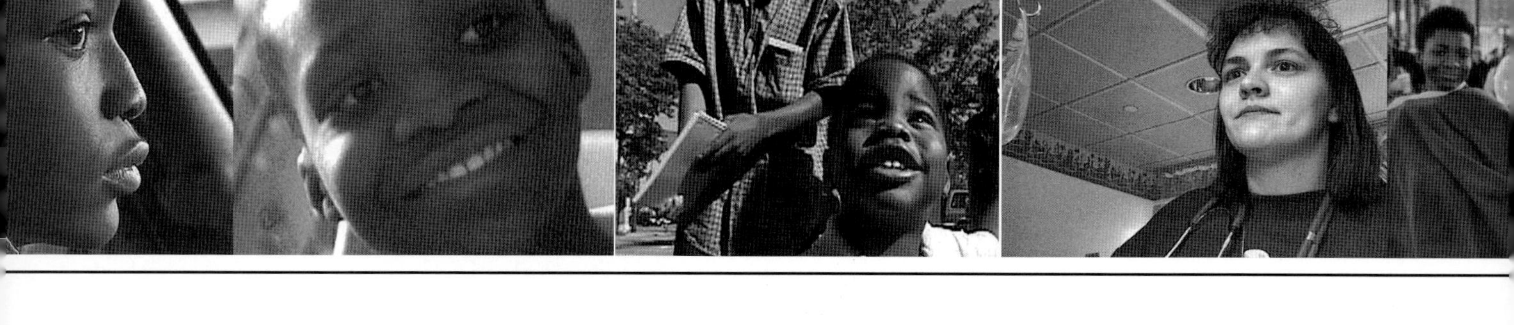

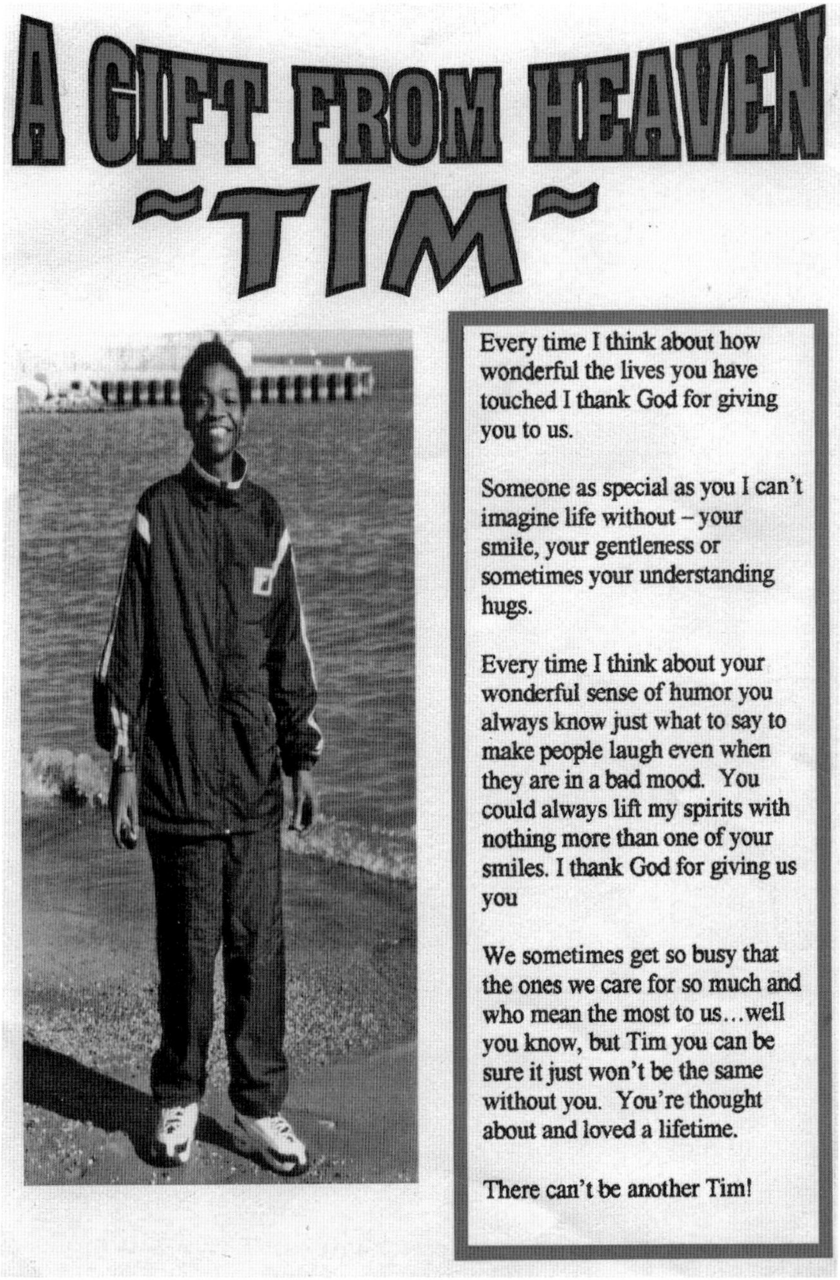

A GIFT FROM HEAVEN

~TIM~

Every time I think about how wonderful the lives you have touched I thank God for giving you to us.

Someone as special as you I can't imagine life without – your smile, your gentleness or sometimes your understanding hugs.

Every time I think about your wonderful sense of humor you always know just what to say to make people laugh even when they are in a bad mood. You could always lift my spirits with nothing more than one of your smiles. I thank God for giving us you

We sometimes get so busy that the ones we care for so much and who mean the most to us…well you know, but Tim you can be sure it just won't be the same without you. You're thought about and loved a lifetime.

There can't be another Tim!

The program cover from Tim's funeral.

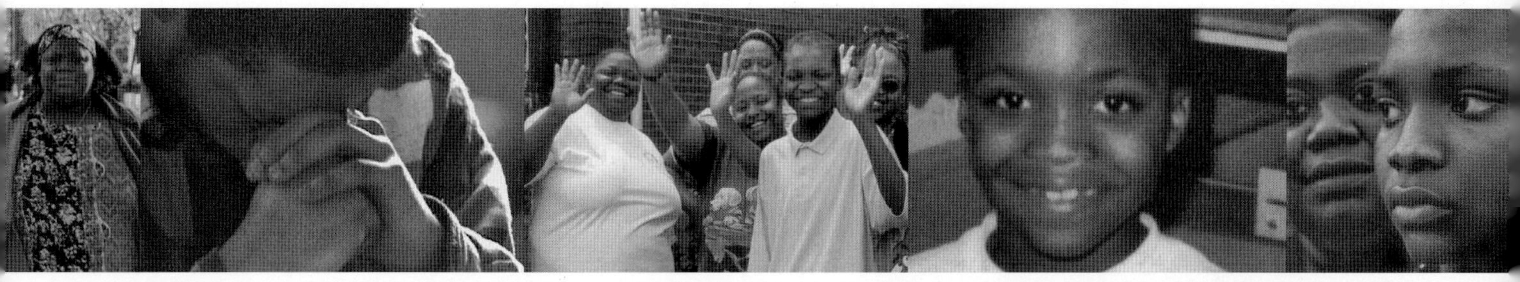

Chapter 4

Alexandra LOUGHEED

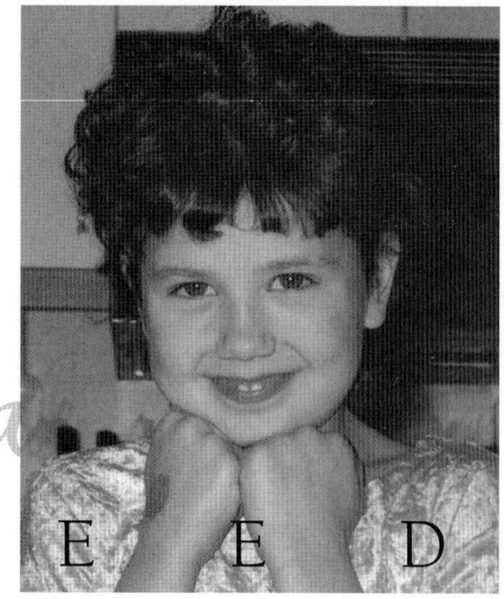

Alex, winner of the "Cutest Personality" award at camp.

scottLOUGHEED

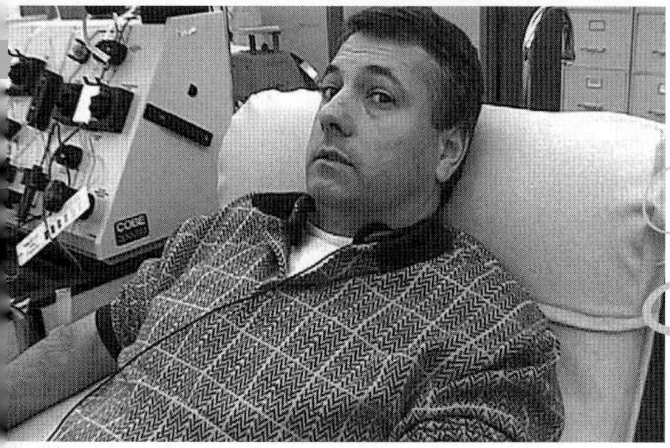

Scott donating his white blood cells to Alex.

During Alexandra's treatment, her father, Scott, donated his bone marrow for a transplant to stem the progress of the disease.

Alex was diagnosed on January 12, 1996. Judy called me: "The doctor thinks that she might have mono and you are going to have to take her to the hospital for a blood test." I took her there and she sat on my lap. I told her, "Honey, I know you aren't going to like this, but they are going to have to give you a 'sticky' (with a needle) to get some blood." Little did I know then how much 'sticky' she was going to have to get.

So they did a blood test. She didn't cry. We took her to McDonalds to get her a Happy Meal. We went home and in two minutes the doctor called. He said, "You need to bring her back in." Judy and I went in. He had tears in his eyes, "I don't know how to tell you this other than to just tell you that your child has leukemia." Honestly, I almost fell on the floor. We took her down to Children's that day. It was the beginning of highs and lows. It was the beginning of hell on earth—if there is a heaven and a hell.

What do I wish I knew on that day? How hard it was going to be.

Knowing what I know now, I would have tried to opt for a more aggressive treatment right from day one. What they told us is that in a couple weeks to a month

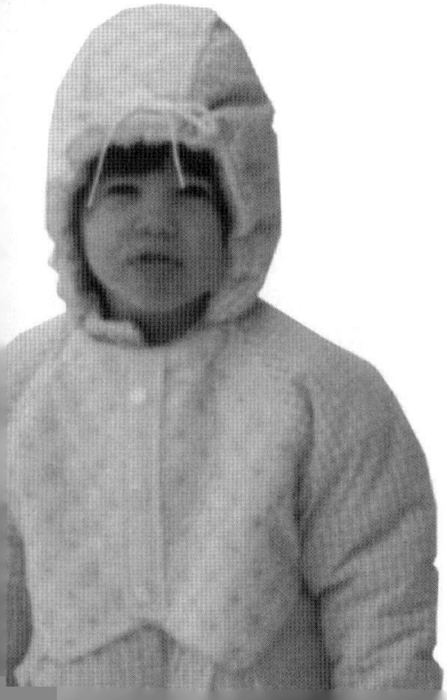

Alex the pink snow bunny.

she'll be in remission. This was January. In April she still wasn't in remission. In May, they finally got her in remission after blitzing her with several doses of heavy, aggressive chemo. She went through a bone marrow transplant, which very few kids (with her condition) go through because they don't have to. After her transplant, she was getting better, got her counts back and started resuming normal life. .

In the summer of '97, we met Steve and Julia. Alex had already been in the battle for eighteen months. She had gotten better. I thought we were out of the woods.

Steve and Julia were great in how the camera was placed. They stayed way out of the way. A lot of the things that went on, you were so wrapped up in what was going on with the child that you just forgot about that—which was good. Some of the things that I saw I don't even remember them filming.

Then in November of 1997, she relapsed. That was a raw point in my life personally because we thought everything was better. You have hopes. It's a road that you go like this (up and down) all the time. November 12, I got a call from my wife. I was in Chicago. Alex went back for her check-up. They took her blood. The leukemia was back.

It devastated my mom. My mom was sixty-one years old at that time. They came down to see Alex. On the way back home, a car ran a stop sign and hit my brother and my mom broadside. My mom was killed. It was absolutely devastating.

(In December 1997, Alex's prognosis was so poor that Judy was advised to make funeral arrangements.) The doctors didn't even tell me. They told my wife, but they hid things from me, which I didn't like. They didn't think I could either handle it or that I would battle it.

One day, Alex was in a clean room. I was looking through some of her charts. They never like to see that either. I read her chart and it said physical therapy—How did it put it?—it was very antiseptic. It said to cancel her physical therapy, child has less than six months to live.

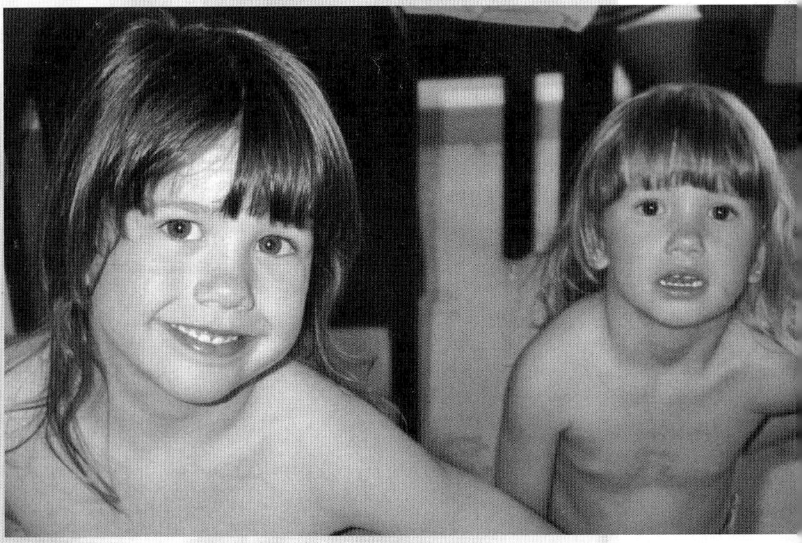

Alex and Jackie, summertime.

I told the doctor there, "Listen, I am a big boy and I should be able to hear that and take that even if I don't like it. Tell me." That's where Paul and I got along so well, because he was wide open. He told me everything. I didn't want to believe the doomsday picture was going to happen, however, he would tell me everything.

Thank the Lord that Paul (Jubinsky) was on service in December. Since it's a teaching hospital, they rotate and you get a doctor of the month—resident of the month.

Alex went through a period of time where she was getting continuous platelets,

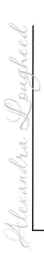

Dr. Paul Jubinsky.

getting blood transfusions, because whatever the medicine was that they gave her, it was eating away at her insides so she was vomiting blood all the time.

I said, "Judy, we can't do this. I don't want to kill my child trying to cure her." Paul had said there are other options we could go to and try. He was able to find a treatment that put her in remission in March of '98.

(That spring, Alex began attending school again, and that summer, she went to Camp Friendship for young cancer patients.)

She stayed in remission till around October '98. She kind of got back, but not normal. When you go through the kind of stuff they put in these kids for aggressive cancer, she would have never been back to what she was. Normal became a different plane.

After she relapsed in late 1998, Alexandra went through more treatment to bring the leukemia under control. In January 1999, an aggressive fungus invaded first her sinuses, then her bone marrow, destroying any chance of restoring her immune function.

Paul told me, "If this is a fungal infection, I don't think Alex will get through this. I really don't. I am just letting you know that. There is a possibility we're sliding down a very slippery slope now." When we brought her home, I knew that there was a probability, a very, very high percentage that she would pass away.

(The Lougheeds took Alex home in February. Her condition continued to deteriorate. Late in May, Scott insisted on asking for more treatment to ease her symptoms, with Dr. Jubinsky's approval.)

Judy and I did have some words where I said, "Listen, we gotta try." I called Paul and I said, "This experimental drug that put her into remission before hasn't been used on her for a year." He said, "You know what, it's worth a try. It didn't give her any toxicity level. Given what we know about this, I think it is a very low risk. It could give her some time. I don't think it will cure her."

So what was my thought going to be? Hey, if you can get your child more time, then it's the best thing to do. It didn't hurt her before. I think that it was a little too late and her body was a little too weak to handle it. Given what I know now, I probably wouldn't have done the things that I did.

But I wanted her to have her last days, for her immune system to fight this a little bit. Maybe it would help her feel better. She wouldn't feel like crap. Everybody was telling me, "You are not doing her any good." All I tried to do was what I thought was good at the time.

Alex at Camp Friendship, a camp for kids fighting cance

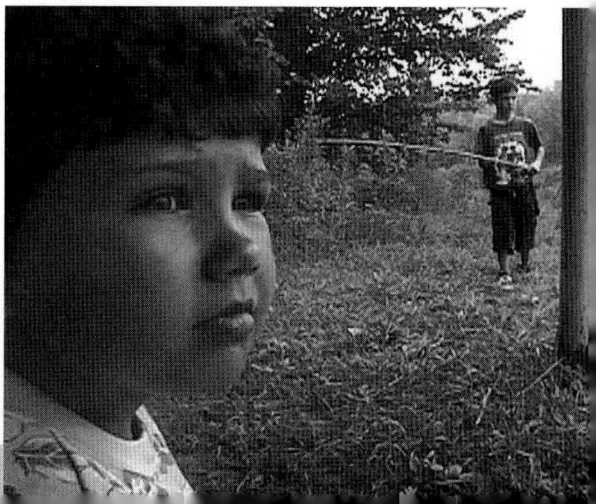

Believe me, when we saw the actual film, it brought raw feelings about it again. In fact, it brought a couple of sleepless nights and I had to get some medication because of panic attacks. We haven't watched any video of Alex at all.

At the very end of the film, I was very upset. I looked like the

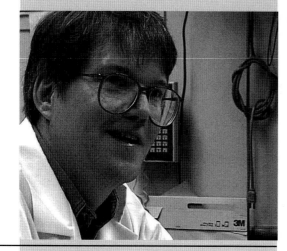

bad guy. I think that I probably upset a lot of people. I was trying to do one thing. I've never given up on anything in my life, and I didn't want to give up on this. As I told Steve and Julia afterward, years after that point I wished I would have changed that. It shows in the movie.

I was looking out for the welfare of my child. She was so terribly sick. I thought it would help her.

Now people say to me, "Are you guys back to normal?" I think, "What the hell do you think?" There is no normalcy when you lose a child, ever. I don't care who you are.

It's changed my whole make-up. It's changed my wife's whole make-up. It's a tremendous strain on a marriage, because you have children that are well.

It totally changed the way my youngest daughter grew up. Jackie doesn't even remember Alex. She sees some of this movie, but she only remembers when she was sick. We lost a lot of focus on Jackie. We shuffled Jackie off to Grandma or other people while we were concentrating on trying to save our other child. It has affected her mentally, emotionally and scholastically. She's not as good a student as she could have been. It's terrible. It's a terrible thing.

Every day I have something that hurts inside that I can't get rid of. For me, the worst times are if I wake up in the middle of the night or right before I wake up in the morning. It's a recurring thing that will probably never leave me.

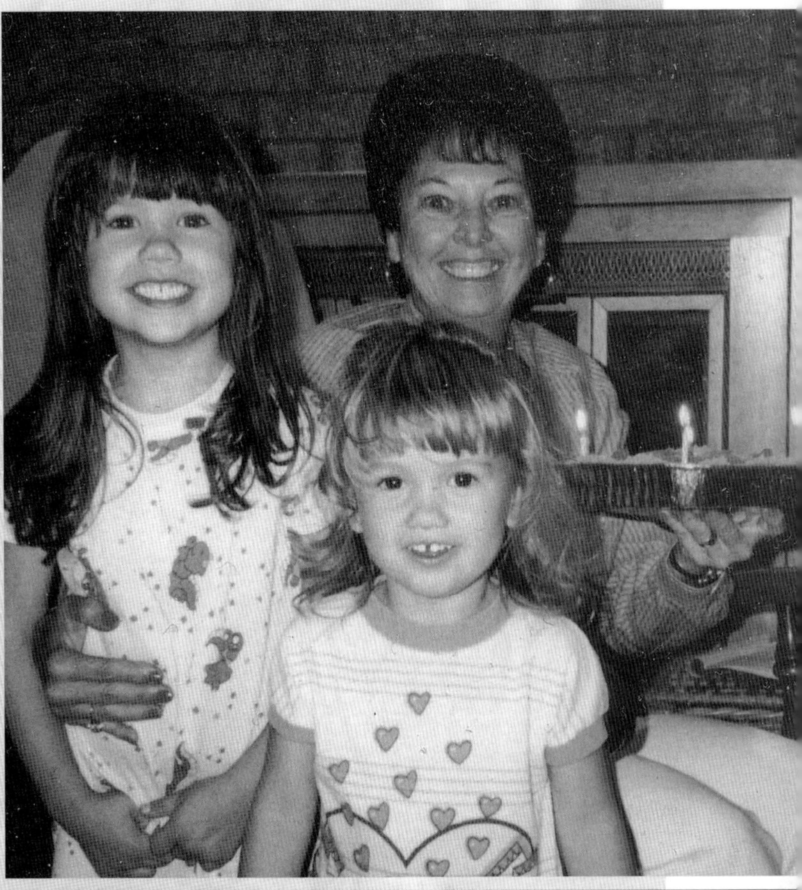

Alex, Jackie and their grandmother, Scott's mother, Evelyn.

Alex was in the hospital eighteen months. When your child is that sick—it's blunt and cold to say so, but you are going to lose your child.

Cancer is not always a death sentence, but if you are that sick they do not have things that can get you through it. If you are in the hospital that much and you survive, it is truly a miracle. All of the children that we became acquainted with and Alex became friends with, every single one of those children died.

I'd like to tell parents to go in with your eyes open. One night in the hospital I was staying with Alex. It was midnight and they were changing her lines because she was on an internal feeding through her C-line. I was lying on the couch looking at all these bottles and asking, "What is that? I've never seen that before." I got up there and looked. It was a new nurse. I saw immediately that this was not Alex's stuff. I didn't make a big deal out of it. I didn't want to get her fired or anything. But it was like, come on, this is life and death.

Judy and I made a pact between us that as long as Alex was in the hospital, either Judy or I was going to stay with her every night that she was there. We held true to that except for one night when Judy's mom came down and stayed with Alex. We had like a free night. If you are in this battle, it affects a relationship. It's probably still affecting our relationship.

I'm not a happy-go-lucky guy. Holidays don't affect me like they used to. It's very bittersweet. We have a child who is thirteen years old that should be enjoying Christmas. It is very bittersweet at this holiday or at Thanksgiving, Easter, you think of the Easter egg hunts. That whole picture, if you put it as a puzzle, there's a big piece missing. You can never go back. The day that we lost her, it was very personal to me. It was on a Saturday. My father was there. The next day was Father's Day. We were sitting there picking out a casket for my daughter. So Father's Day is a horrible holiday for me.

When I see sick children, it's like a knife that goes right in my rib. I'm not a guy that tears up a lot, but I do tear up a lot more than I did before. It's made me more compassionate. We are guarded about trying to be happy. Why should I be happy? I lost a child. Why should I laugh? Believe it or not, initially the first few months I felt guilty if someone told a joke and it was funny. I still joke around, but I used to be crazy joking around with all my friends. I'm not as jovial as I used to be. I'm more serious. It's changed that, maybe for the good. There is no way that we can go back to the way that we lived before and bring it back to today. I think Judy sees different times when she's reflecting upon what could have been. I've done the same. There's no getting over it ever, to certain degrees. The hurt has become less sharp and has turned to a dull pain.

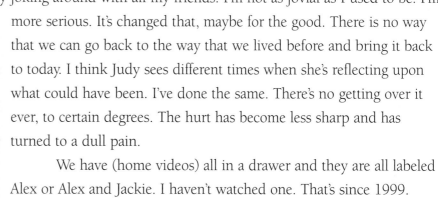

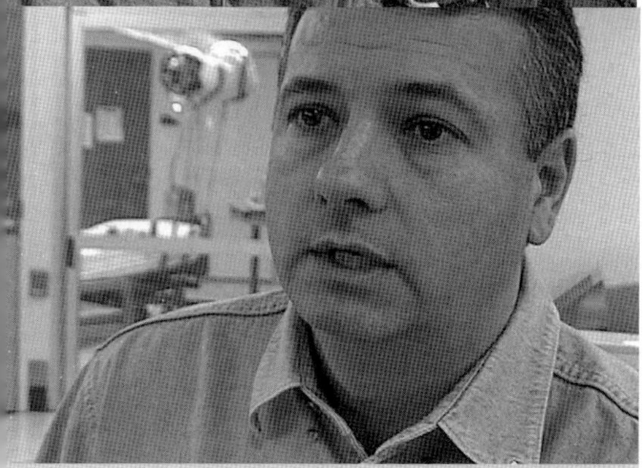

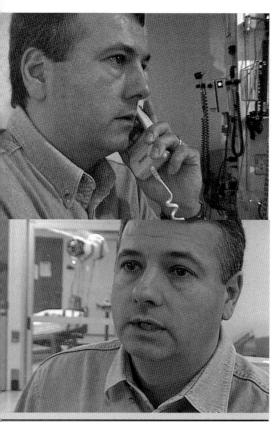

Top:
Scott gets the news that his donated white blood cells have dramatically boosted Alex's ANC.

Bottom:
Scott Lougheed outside of Alex's room in Cincinnati Children's Hospital. Scott and Judy faced excruciating decisions together.

We have (home videos) all in a drawer and they are all labeled Alex or Alex and Jackie. I haven't watched one. That's since 1999. We stopped filming. I actually put the video camera away when she got really sick. It's like you almost want to block it out because it is still so raw.

Alex was Judy's and my first child. You know how the first child you have a lot of photos and you have the video and you tape an hour of that child just lying in the crib doing nothing?

Alex had my hair color and kind of my personality. She was very mischievous. She touched a lot of lives. I guess that's more important than anything. I just wish she would have been able to touch more lives. She never really was able to do some of the things that children get to do at her age. She never really rode a bike. We were terrified. She had a bike with training wheels. Everything scared us and it affected the way that we brought Jackie up too. We were more protective.

I don't know how some of the days we were able to get

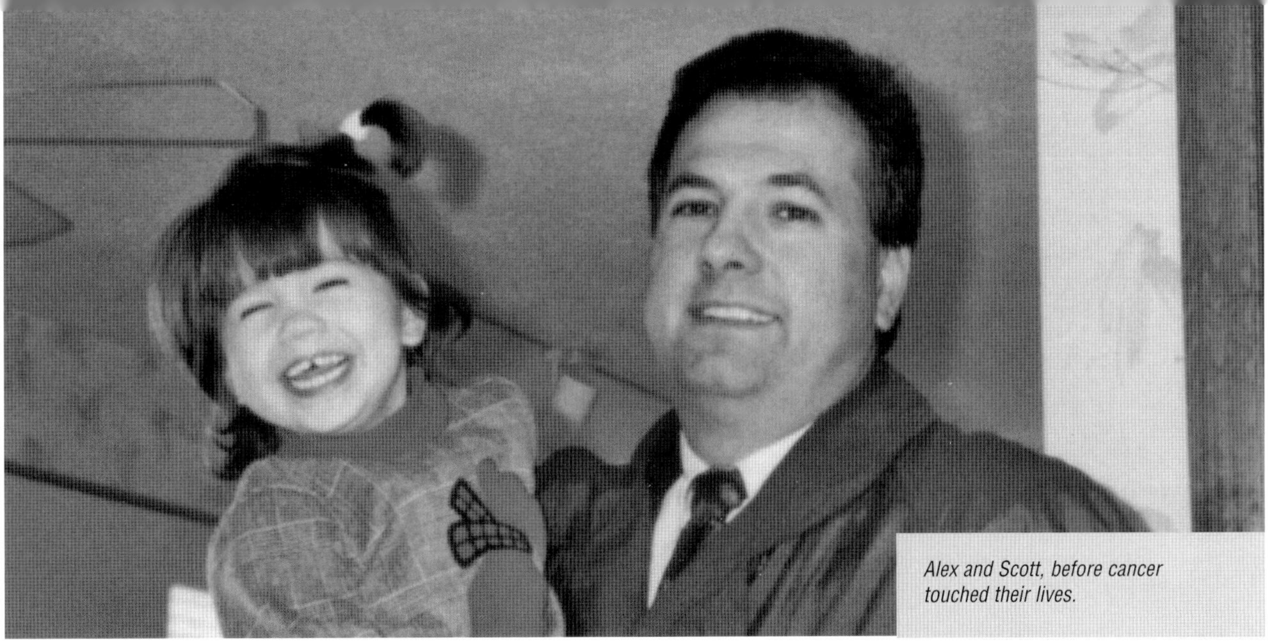

Alex and Scott, before cancer touched their lives.

through it or how some of those families were able to get through it. You just do. I had a friend who came to Alex's funeral. He said to me later, "Scott, I don't know how you did what you did." I gave the eulogy. I told him I don't know how I did it either. When I even think about it today, I don't know how I did it.

If there is divine intervention, it has really affected my faith too. This is hard to say because I don't like to talk about religion. I'm not sure there is a God. I grew up in a small farming community in Northwest Ohio. I went to Sunday School every Sunday. We were Methodist and were brought up to believe in God. This whole thing rocked me.

The thing that I look at in the overall experience is that I miss my daughter and I wish she were here. Maybe she is in spirit. I don't want to say that I don't hope that I'm going to see her. I hope I do, to touch her again.

Many people think you could get over it, but I don't know how anyone can get over it. I don't know how other parents have dealt with the loss of a child, but it's affected my life in very dramatic ways. Unless you have been there, it's different. If someone has lost a child due to a car accident, it's different. If someone has lost a child due to a drug overdose, it's different. We lost a child and we watched her suffer for many, many months, and it's heart wrenching.

I lost my mom, but it's a different hurt. It's a bitter pill when I lost my daughter. It's like if I could take this size hurt *(he holds his arms wide)* when I lost my mom, when I lost Alex the hurt was the size of this room. It's something that is a part of you that you lose that you are so enamored with.

The thing that helps me in some ways is that we are not the only ones that have gone through this. Five different families and for every one of them there has been a tragedy. You just wish that that did not have to happen. I learned from all those kids, not just Alex, down at Children's. It can

Alex at Disneyworld Mickey has nothing on her!

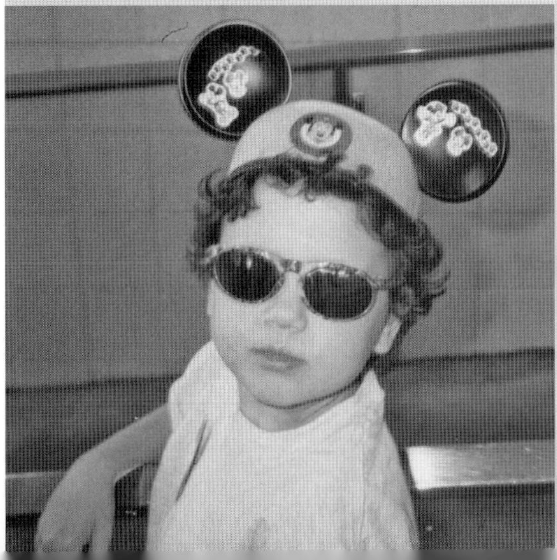

be as bleak as anybody can see and these kids were just carrying on. Bald headed, looked like death warmed over—you learn that these kids are tough kids.

Alex never went to intensive care. You would see Justin (Ashcraft) was up and down from ICU. If I think I had a hard time, when did they surrender? It's like maybe if I were in that situation with them, maybe I would have surrendered earlier. You don't know when it's their time. You are going to fight for their lives and it's a war—never surrender. I don't know that I ever asked Alex or that my wife ever came to terms to saying that. How do you ask her if she wanted to die?

judyLOUGHEED

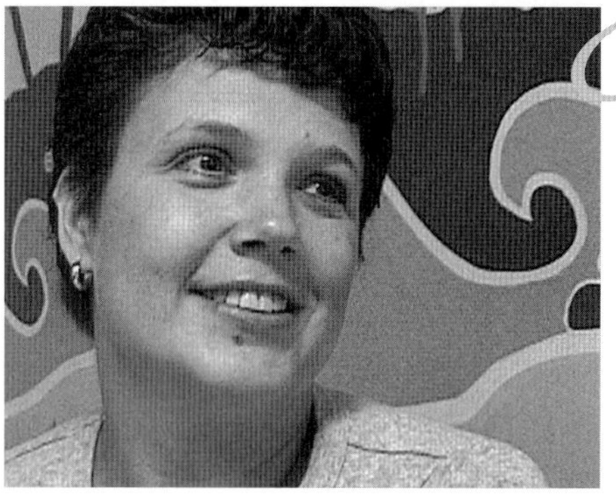

Judy Lougheed expresses concern about sending Alex to camp.

Judy Lougheed and her husband shared responsibility for staying with Alexandra each time she was hospitalized.

I stayed during the week. Scott came on the weekends. I left. I did the laundry. Went to the grocery store, cooked for the week. Came back at the end of the weekend and traded places. That's how we did it. We had to. We had a kid at home and a kid at the hospital. My mom would come down occasionally and sit with Alex and we'd have some time alone together.

I don't think we ever made a decision in the hospital without conferring with one another. They would give us an opinion on what we should do, they would leave and we would sit there for a day. Whatever it took. Discuss the pros, discuss the cons, and basically make our decision from there.

Alex was very brave person. I don't know if I could be like that in the situation she was in. There were times when I wanted to break down, wring somebody's neck, kick somebody. She never faltered through any of that.

She would be so sick but she'd always have a smile for everybody. She always had a hug for everybody. She would walk around that hallway with Scott pushing the pole (with her IV bags), stopping in everybody else's window, looking in, smiling and waving to them. She'd be the goodwill ambassador for the floor.

I just feel sorry for Alex. She was just five years old when she was diagnosed and almost nine when she died. Those are great childhood years, and what did she get to do? Nothing. She got to lie in a hospital bed or in a bed at home and have IVs hooked up to her. There were times when she'd go into remission, we'd go to the beach and things like that, but still it wasn't much of a childhood. Alex did not even know what it was to be a kid.

She had a great singing voice for her age. She was very artistic, very good with people. I think if she would have stayed alive, she would have amounted to something really great.

Since she is gone, I get so bitter about things. I see all these people on TV who leave their kids at home while they go out and they look for drugs. You hear horror stories on the news (and think), "Why is this bully allowed to live when someone so sweet, who could have done so much

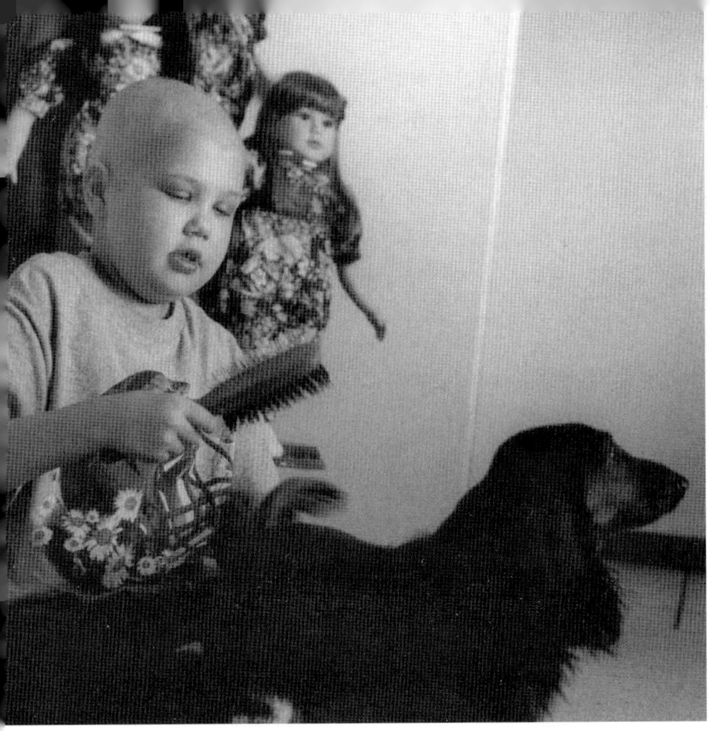

Alex combing Dylan, a palliative care pet.

good for this world, why is she allowed to die?"

I was reading the newspaper (about a new cancer treatment). I stopped it and went on to something else. I don't care. It's too late for us. And that's sad that I have that attitude, because I should be hoping that kids in the future can make it. But right now I am not at that point. It's like that friend who called me the other day to get together so I can see how much her 11-year-old has grown.

There were some days that are worse than others. I don't know what set it off. There were days when I didn't feel like doing anything. I just wanted to sit around the house and mope and feel sorry for myself. I wanted everybody else to feel sorry for me.

Scott deals with things in a different way than I do. We were going through that photo album (from Steve and Julia). I was just so happy to see pictures of Alex, and they were beautiful pictures. I was glad that somebody remembered her. And he would look at the pictures and immediately it was like, "Oh God, why did this happen to her?" I was looking at it as a good thing and he was looking at it as a very sad thing. It brings me down. I know he doesn't do that on purpose. That's just his way of dealing with it.

(Recalling Scott's insistence on taking Alexandra in for treatment in her last days:) Maybe that's why he gets sad. At the end, she wanted to stay home and be comfortable and he was forcing her to go the strange hospital bed and get chemo and eat their strange food and nobody wants to do that when they don't feel good.

We did find a church that we really liked. At that time it felt like we really needed a church. We went a few times. We actually started feeling better. I don't know what happened. That feeling just went away. Something in me didn't want to go anymore. I figured that if I wanted to talk to God or if I wanted to pray, there was no reason I couldn't do it anywhere. A part of me, I guess, felt angry at the Lord. I don't feel guilty at all for not going. I don't lose sleep over it at all.

(Many parents report sensing the presence of a child who has passed away.) The only time I did was right after she died. Scott had gone somewhere out of town. I did not sleep well that entire weekend. I kept hearing footsteps through this house. I kept hearing doors shut. I kept hearing cabinets open and shut. It was freaking me out. I was actually scared.

During the next day I didn't hear anything. Or if I did, it wasn't as bad.

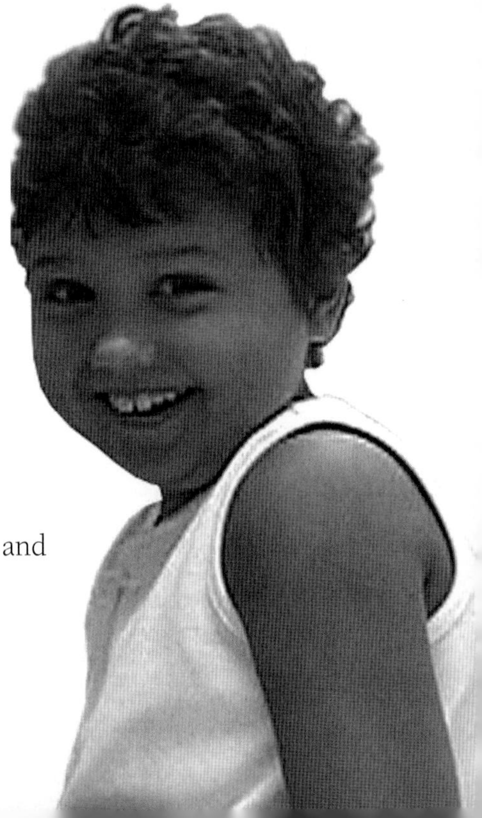

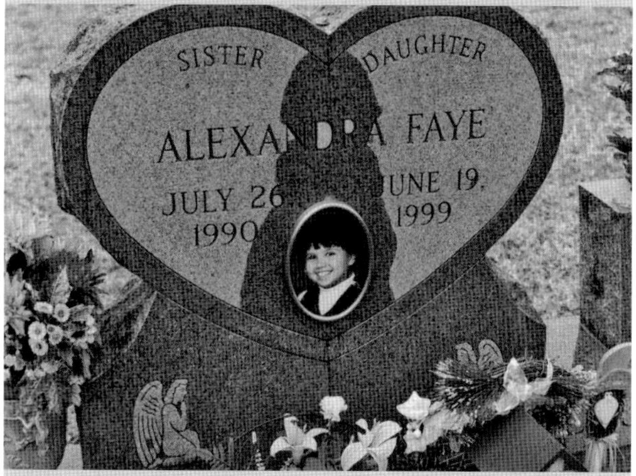

Alex's gravestone, after an Autumn rain.

During the day, I started thinking about it and I said, "Alex? If that's you then that's fine, but you have to realize that mommy's here by herself and it's scaring her. If you want to stay here, that's great, but could you do it in a less scary way? Because you are really freaking me out (laughing). Don't shut doors, do something else." I said that kind of over and over again.

Scott and I used to hear music come up through the vents in the bedroom. We could not figure out what music it was. We'd be lying there in the middle of the night, wide awake listening. Neither one of us knew the other one was awake. We both heard it for days and days.

One big thing is that neither one of us is afraid to die now. I know that I have my beautiful daughter waiting for me. I believe that you have to be the best person you can be. Everybody sins, everybody does. But if you are trying to be the best person you can be and you honestly feel bad about the bad things you do, I think you are going to go to heaven. I am looking forward for my beautiful daughter being there to greet me as I walk through those pearly gates.

brittanyLOUGHEED

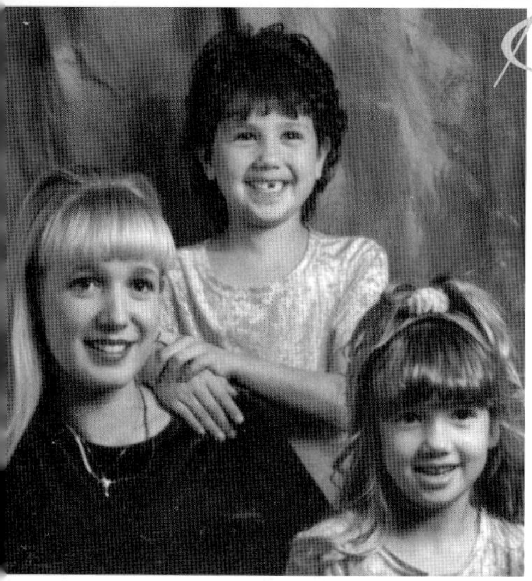
Brittany, Alexandra, & Jaclyn, the Lougheed sisters.

Brittany Lougheed, who was sixteen when Alex was diagnosed, is Judy's first daughter, whom Scott adopted after he and Judy married. Brittany had moved out of her parents' home by the time filming began.

The day they found out Alex had cancer she had a spot on her face that was all dry and we thought she had allergies, like the rest of the family. I remember I was in the bathroom blow drying my hair when my mom walked upstairs and she was standing there in the doorway and she didn't say anything. Her eyes were all red and she had been crying. I'm thinking, *What's going on here?*

"Well we just came from the doctor. Alex has leukemia. She has cancer." I didn't even know what to say. What do you mean she has cancer? She is only five years old. She can't have cancer. They said she had to go to the hospital that day, right then.

I wanted to give her something like a stuffed animal, something from her big sister. I remember when she was getting ready to leave I was sitting there on the couch and I was crying. I was upset and she just looked at me and she was concerned about me, if I was going to be okay, and she just waved at me like that as she was leaving. I see her sitting there waving. I see that all the time. That's just a picture of her that I can't forget.

I knew she was most protective with my mom. She was like that with all of us.

After her final hospitalization in 1999, Alex was sent home for hospice care.

At first I was thrilled Alex was coming home, didn't understand what it meant that someone was in hospice. I kept asking my mom questions. I wasn't in meetings with them (the doctors). How come nobody's happy that she's coming home?

When she was in the hospital, everything was normal, you wouldn't even think there was a problem there. But when you've got hospice here and a portable bed in the living room, this isn't normal.

I didn't think this was Alex's last few weeks. They didn't want to share with me the details of what was going on. What made me angry was that they knew that I wanted to know what was going on. When I would hear them talk about something I didn't know about, I would get angry. "What is going on? Why don't you tell me things? You know, I'm getting sick of guessing what's going on here."

The parents, I think they should talk about all of it. It's not fair to the other child to only know bits and pieces and leave the bad stuff out. If something's going bad and the parents are thinking, *Well, maybe these could be her last days, shouldn't they know that too?* I think so.

It's so hard to read what the both of them are thinking. I think my dad's always been guywise, like, "Nothing is going to happen; no matter what goes on, nothing is going to happen to her, she'll be fine." More like blocking out. I think he did that too, just like I did.

I think my mom, having to deal with it every single day and every minute of the day and having to take phone calls from the doctors and listening to everything that people were telling her, she maybe felt a few more doubts because reality was pushed more on her than on me and my dad.

(Judy) was tired all the time, constantly tired, she was more like—I want to say moody, but her patience was wearing thin because she was dealing with so much else and you bring something else on her and it's kind of like, "I don't want to deal with this right now, I have so much else to worry about."

She really didn't have much time to do anything. It's not like you can ask the neighbor, "Can you come over and watch Alex while I go to the grocery?" It was every hour of the day that Alex needed medication, and you can't just have anyone coming over and sitting with her. Somebody's gotta know how to take care of her, and with my dad being gone a lot, my mom barely had time to go to the grocery store in between medicines. She had time to do the laundry basically. It was just wearing her out.

During Alex's illness, Brittany graduated from high school, and moved in with her grandmother, enrolled in college and got a job.

My first quarter wasn't bad; it was

Judy and Jackie Lougheed at home.

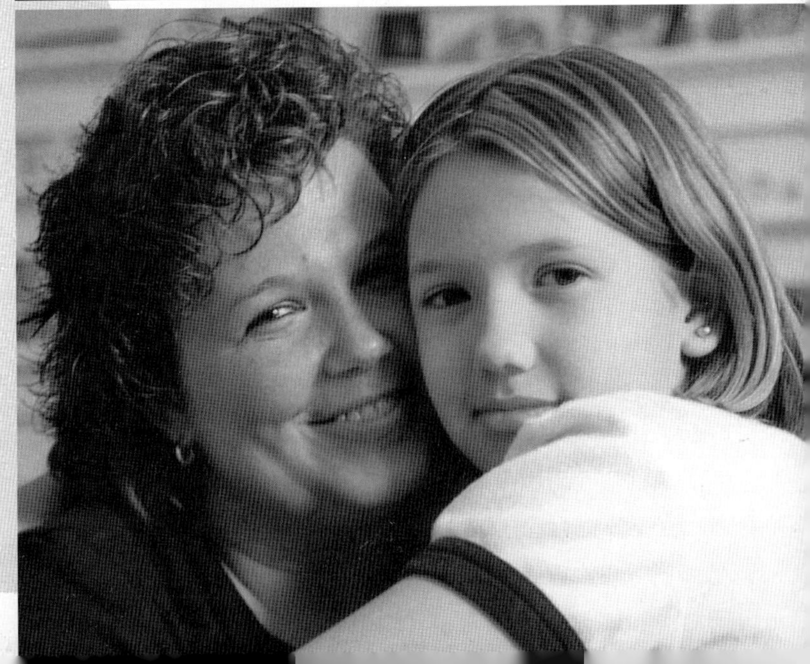

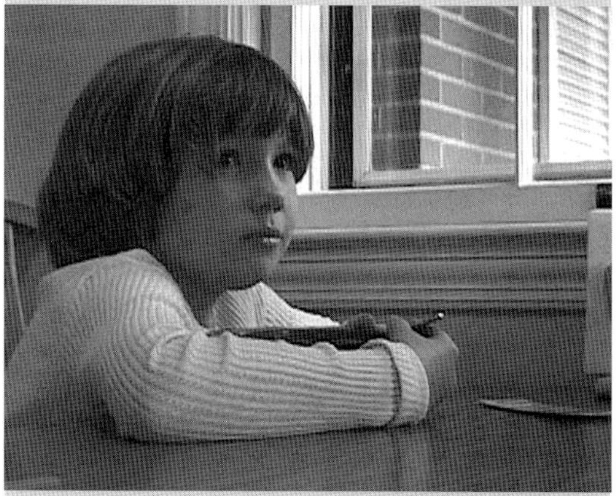

Alex's little sister Jackie at home. Like so many siblings, she was sometimes pushed to the margins, despite her parents' best efforts.

getting used to it, it was the basics. Second quarter was after Alex relapsed and I didn't do very good second quarter. Actually I was very lucky to get the grades that I did get, because, honestly, I didn't work hard at all. I didn't study like I should have; I didn't do homework like I should have. Second quarter I didn't even want to get up and go to school. Then when I was in school I didn't want to be there, so I left early and came over here. I didn't want to go to work because I didn't want to be away from her and when I did have to go to school all day and then go to work from school, it was like I shouldn't be doing this, this isn't fair, I should be spending time with my sister.

I think the relationship between the two of us changed a lot after she got sick. I was big sister, I was in charge, and after she got sick I didn't want to be like that anymore. I just wanted to twirl her.

She was smart, extremely smart and I take some credit for that because when she was little, I always wanted to do the little flash cards with her and stuff. It's kind of like having a little pet.

She knew anything any kid could possibly learn in kindergarten. The teacher told my mom that she didn't know what she was going to teach Alex because Alex knew everything already. She knew her phone number and her address and her birthday and she could count to 100. She was only five and she could count to 100. She knew all of her colors and she knew all of her shapes.

I felt bad about Jackie. We could have worked a little bit more with her but it was like she was the second one.

I remember dad going into (Alex's) room to talk to her just a couple weeks before she died. He was kind of going in to make his peace with her. He was sitting in there and he could barely speak because he was so upset and he was crying, and she said, "Dad, it's going to be okay." And he's going, "Here's my eight-year-old telling me it's going to be all right." You don't know what to say when she says something like that 'cause it's like, "Okay, I guess it will be if you say so."

She would sit there and listen to him just because she knew that he needed to say that to her for him to feel better, and if that would make him feel better then she would sit there and listen, and that was fine and he would be all right.

I look back and of course I have all these things I want to say to her still and it's like I can't say them now, at least not directly to her.

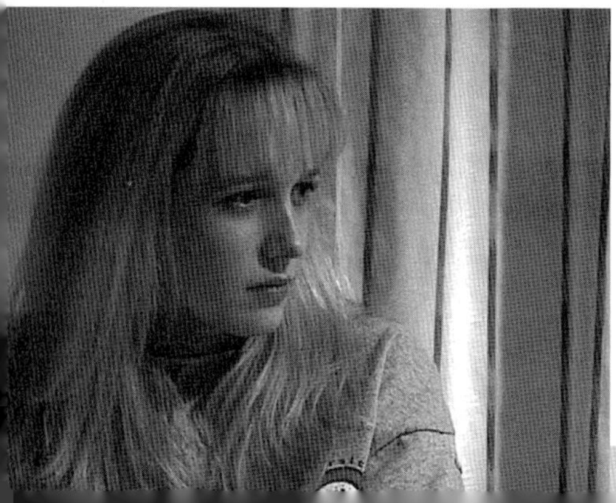

She told my mom one time when I came over here, "I wish that Brittany came over to see me one time," and mom is like, "She comes over all the time." Alex said, "She comes over to see everyone else, too. I want her to come over here just to see me." When I came over to take care of her that night, I was in her room and Jackie came in and wanted to play cards with me. I said, "You know what, normally any other time

Brittany in Alex's room at Cincinnati Children's Hospital.

I would play cards with you, but tonight I cannot play cards with you. I am Alex's nurse, because I came here just for Alex, just to see her, just to take care of her, so I cannot play cards with you tonight." And I looked over and saw Alex's little smile, 'cause she knew that I was over there just for her. I was glad that I was able to do that.

I'm not a mushy person. I don't tell people how I feel and I kind of hide my emotions. I felt if I started getting mushy with her and telling her all these things, she would know that there was something wrong. "Why is she doing that now? She doesn't say things like that, she doesn't act like that. Something must be wrong if she's doing all this now.'

When I look back, she's not here now, I should have just said it. When I look at it now, it wouldn't have mattered. I was thinking that if everyone else stayed strong and she wanted to bad enough, that she was going to live, no matter what happened. But that wasn't the case. Nobody gave up on her. She didn't give up on herself, you know? She just couldn't take it any more. And I think, well, it would've been an indication that I was giving up on her if I had said that to her. But I should've said it anyway, because she's not here anymore.

It all depends on what kind of relationship you have had up till then. If you've always been the kind of person to constantly tell people how you feel and constantly tell them how much they mean to you, then yeah, you can pretty much tell them whatever you wanted and the kid would pretty much think that was normal. But if you've had the relationship that you hold everything back, and then just all of a sudden you're just spilling everything out, it might scare them because it's not normal.

I took an English class in school and they asked what writing means to us. Writing means to me that I don't say things that I feel, but I can write them.

(Brittany wrote a private letter addressed to Alex after her death. She has never shared it with anyone.) That letter is everything that I wanted to say to her over the three years when she was sick. It took me ten minutes to write it all down on paper. I thought maybe if I got it all out, maybe then she would just know. It's not like she can sit there at the cemetery and read it, but maybe if I can get it all out and think it in my head, she will just know.

Ever since she died, I've had this strange feeling. I walk through the house and, obviously she's not here like she's always been, but I don't feel like she's gone. I said to Mom, maybe she doesn't want me to feel like she's gone. Just because her body isn't here and I can't see her doesn't mean that she has left us.

I want her in front of me. I want to see her, you know? Ever since she was little, I thought, I want to teach her how to drive. I want to give her advice about her boyfriends and all that, and I'm going to help her decide what kind of clubs she should do, should she be a cheerleader. That's why I'm going miss her, because I won't be able to do all that stuff with her. I have this picture of her when she was four or five and she is so pretty, I could just imagine her when she was seventeen or eighteen. She would've been so beautiful.

I think she's helped me see what is really important, not just what everyone else thinks is important. My family is really important, but I never realized that before. I just assumed they would always be there, and now that they're not, you don't know what can happen. You just have to decide what is important to you and you have to show those people that they are important to you.

I think she has helped me be more responsible, because with my parents having to deal with everything, I didn't want them to have to worry about me. So it was kind of my personal goal to be a responsible person. Actually, since she passed away, I'm trying to be more honest, 'cause she can see everything I'm doing. Now she can see everything and hear everything I'm saying and I don't want her to see me telling a lie. So I'm going to not disappoint her.

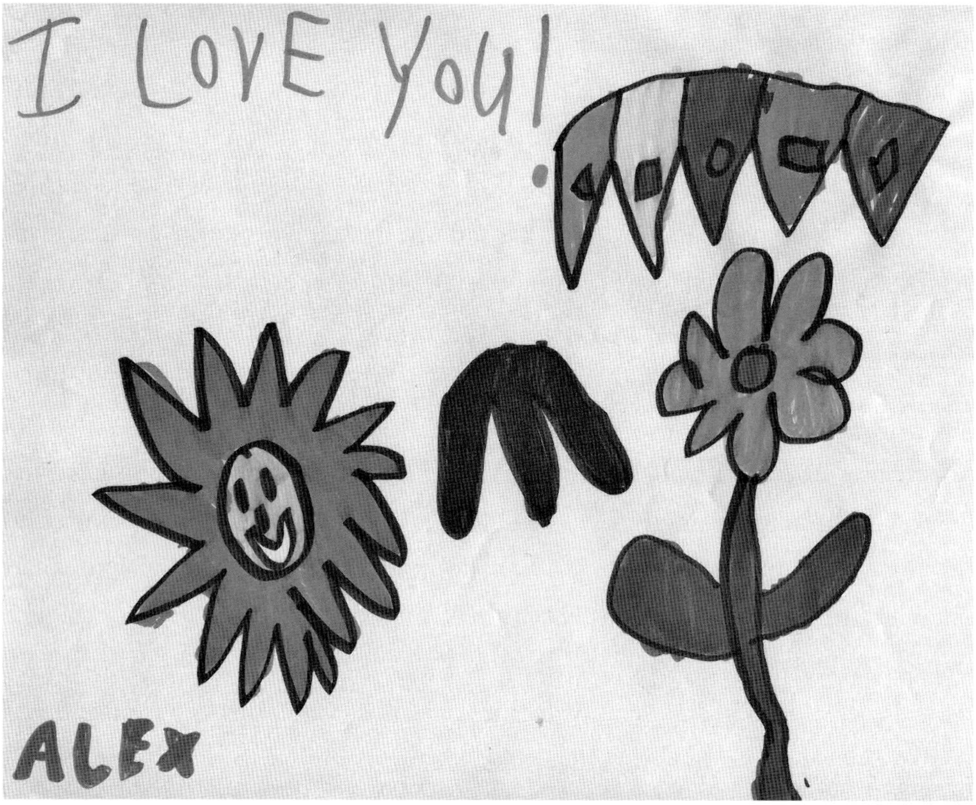

Alex's artwork

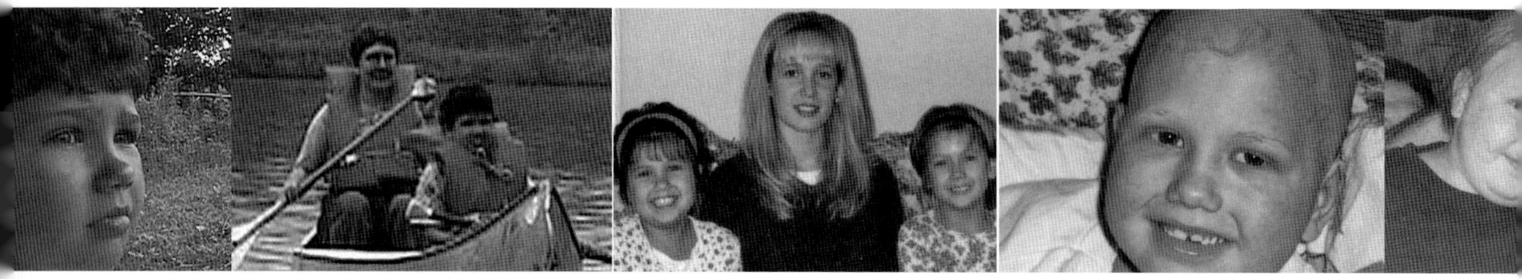

Filmmakers' Journal

Steven: The first day of filming was July 4, 1997, when we visited Judy, Alex, Jackie Lougheed, and Gramma June, at their home north of Cincinnati. Scott was working that day. Alex and Jackie were racing around the backyard on their big wheels, as you see in the film. I couldn't believe the energy these two little half-pints had, how fast they would get going on these things, and how they totally crashed into each other with such complete abandon and joy. It was the raw energy of youth in full effect. I ran around with the camera, keeping it at their eye level, and it was then that years of working in schools, making movies with kids, came in handy because the footage did seem to capture some of their energy. I'm proud of how the camera kind of flies through the air in that scene. And I'm glad that the last shot of the entire film goes back to that first day of filming, as Alex races away from the camera on her Big Wheel.

Julia: But Alex was not just a cute, appealing little girl. Take another look at that shot of Alex, as she responds to Steve asking, "Are you exhausted?" She says, "Nope!" But you can see layers, more layers of all she has been through, layers of thought, worry, pain, flash across her face. Her hospice nurse Lynn put it well: "She had those eyes that could just penetrate your soul." Whenever Alex asked, "How are you?" she really wanted to know. She listened. She was almost always cheery, positive, trying to crack jokes. She was an old soul.

Alex was also an amazing artist, an aspect I am so sorry got cut from the final film. She had an innate sense of design and color, and her drawings were chosen by the hospital as Christmas cards. As she declined, and the chemo and various interventions really were getting to her, it was just tragic to watch her draw, her hands shaking and tentative. It was as if cancer were taking parts of her, piece by piece. It broke my heart.

The Lougheed nuclear family was utterly mobilized behind Alex, her mom and dad. It was inspiring to watch. The Lougheeds did heroic things to save that girl.

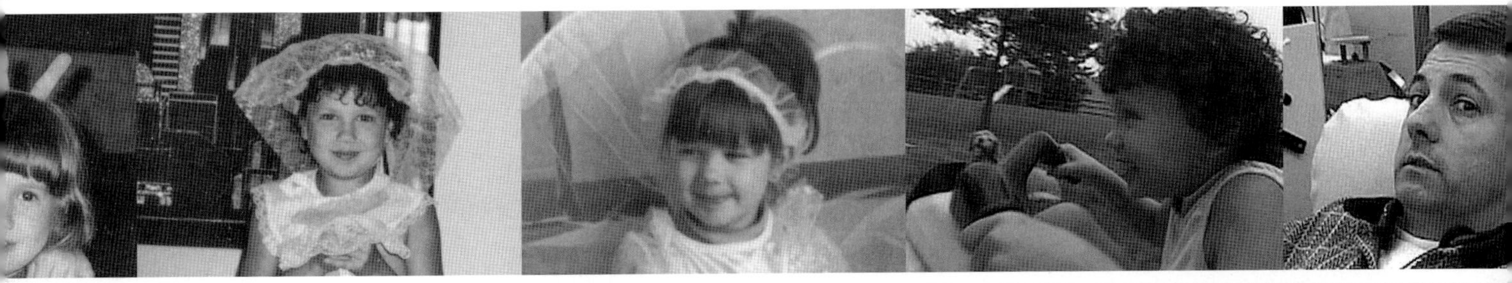

Chapter 5

Alex FIELDS

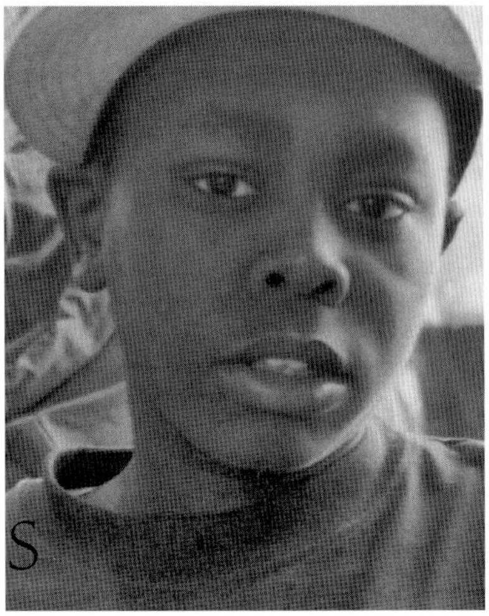

Al Fields, on his thirteenth birthday.

reginaFIELDS

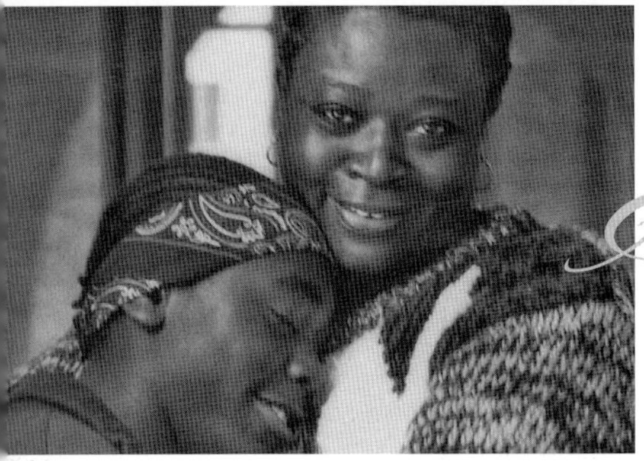

A single mother, Regina saw her son Alex through treatment for non-Hodgkin's lymphoma while working full-time at the nursing home where she is still employed. She also is raising three of Al's young cousins.

Al and Regina after a successful follow-up checkup at Cincinnati Children's. For a cancer survivor, going back to a hospital for a follow-up visit almost always creates anxiety.

The first thing I thought about (on the day of diagnosis) was death. When he said cancer I was like, "Oh, my baby is going to die." However, Al took it in stride. He said, "Oh, Mama, we can do it; we can do it."

They're pretty good doctors here, 'cause they really saved my child's life. 'Cause my child could have left me. Fred Huang was his doctor. Fred will always be in my heart. They will always be in my heart. He saved my baby.

Dr. Huang stuck with him when he had his tantrums. He told him "No." He told him "Yes." He really was a good doctor. His profession suits him. He loves the kids. He spoils them. He's not one of those doctors that only talks to the parents. He talks to the kids and breaks it down to their level too.

The first thing I said after my reaction to the diagnosis was, "I don't do drugs." I couldn't understand why my child was sick. Cancer ran on his daddy's side of the family. His dad's mother had cancer and is in remission. None on my side. That's why they want to know both sides of the family's medical history. I didn't know that she had it till Al had it.

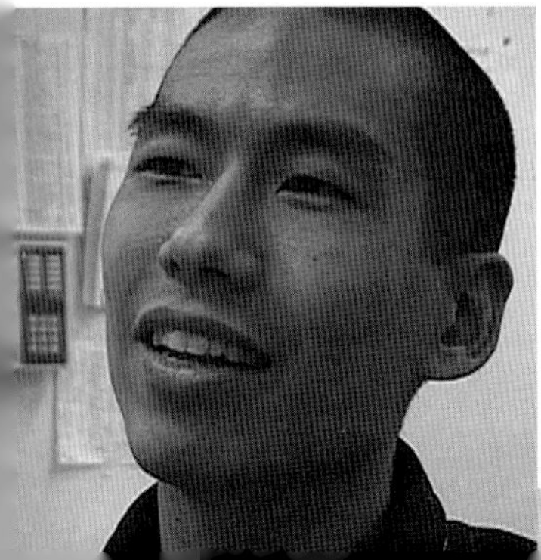

Dr. Fred Huang, Al's oncologist. Regina joked that she would someday marry Dr. Fred.

I would have liked to have known he was sick sooner. Al has always been short and chubby like. Then he started losing weight and getting tall. I thought he was just getting taller. Then one night he came home and said, "Mama, I can't breathe; Mama, I can't breathe." So I took him over there to Children's Hospital. I would have liked to have known the signs of it. I had taken him to the doctor for his check-up four months before. The doctor said that he was fine.

Then in June he got sick. They said, "We have got to call this doctor and see if this will be okay if we can check him out." I said, "No, you don't need to call his doctor. I'm his doctor. I'm his mama and you have my permission." I told them I had just taken him to the doctor four months ago. The man said his chest was all right.

When they took an x-ray, you couldn't even see his lungs. It was just cloudy. The mass was on the lungs. It wasn't inside the lungs; it was outside going up, blocking him from breathing. When they did the biopsy on him, they couldn't do it anywhere except on his neck. He had to be awake. They couldn't put him under because it would have killed him. They had to do it with him awake. When he laid on that bed, the top surgeon at Children's did that.

The hardest part for me was the hospital part. He was there for a month because they had to shrink the tumor first. He had three days of radiation and chemo. They couldn't start chemo till they shrunk it.

I can say that he didn't get too sick with the chemo. He was kind of weak when his (white blood cell) counts were down. He didn't get too sick, like throwing up or mouth sores. He got the sores once. They were giving him the chemo, that was the shots. It put a blood clot in his leg. That come because they couldn't find no veins in his arms. They put a shunt in. They shot the chemo in his thigh with his leg up and it caused a blood clot. That's the only thing that didn't go right. He didn't go through the throwing up.

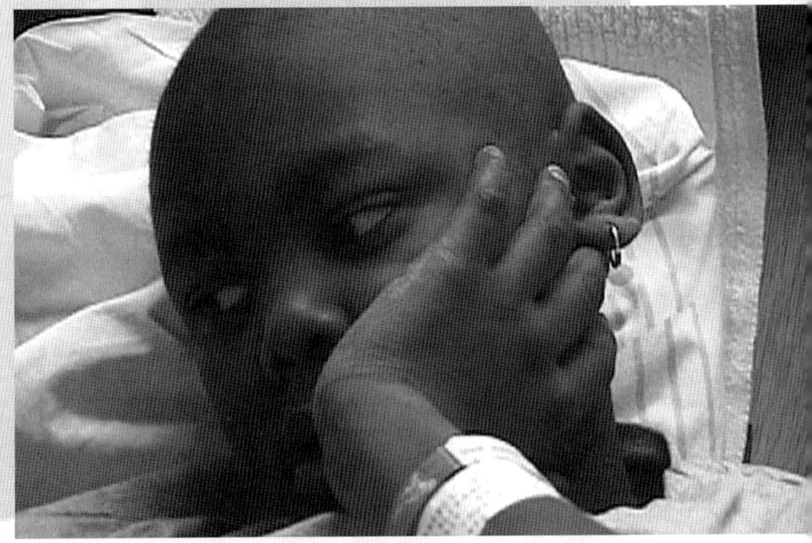
Al feeling lousy.

(A sequence in the film shows Dr. Huang explaining to Al why he cannot go to camp because he is due for a round of chemo.) Al, he accepted it. I explained to him that it was either life or play. He knew that Dr. Huang had never lied to him or never hid nothing from him. They always said there will be another trip. His counts were real low then. If they had been 15,000 or something like that, then he could have skipped the chemo for that time. That day he needed blood. There was no question about it.

There were doctors who didn't always tell you everything. One time, Al had just come from the clinic and was running this high fever. When he got this other times, it

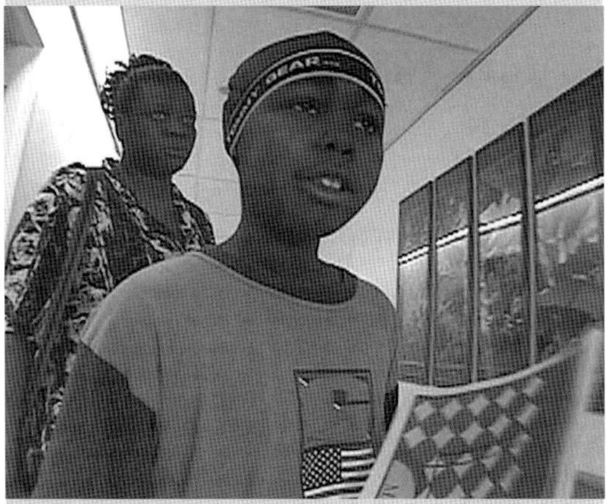

Al and Regina on the move. Even though he was only eleven years old, Al got to know the hospital like the back of his hand.

because he had infection. Another time he had the high fever was when he had the blood clot. So I took him to emergency again.

This foreign doctor came out and told me they were going to have to have surgery, that his leg would have to be cut open. On chemo, they can catch anything. The doctor came out and I said, "You said surgery? Let me get this right. Why? Because it looks just like a blood clot to me. That is the symptoms of a blood clot." I can't think of that man's name, but what he said is going to stick with me every day. He was pediatrics emergency. I was cussing up a storm. I asked questions, but I didn't yell at people.

He said, "We are going to bring another doctor in here from the floor." Dr. Huang came in that night to check on him. I told him that he (the other doctor) was going to cut my baby's leg. He said, "No, he's not."

Another resident, I think her name was Joan, she sat down with us. They had my baby on oxygen in intensive care. She came to me. I'm sitting there watching him sleep and breathe. She explained to me that they were going to do radiation on him. It took three doctors and six nurses just to take my baby to give the radiation. No one really bothered me except that emergency doctor. Everybody else was straightforward. You know, they come in there talking about big words, but they broke it down. I had the medical book, and I looked it up to see what they were talking about.

It was like hell (when Al was hospitalized). It was going to work, coming here (to the hospital), going to work, coming here. It was like an everyday thing. I didn't have time for myself. I was mostly there at night. Everybody was in bed. In the morning, I'd leave after he ate breakfast to go home, to go to bathe and go back to the hospital till it was time to go to work.

They tried to give me this room away from him (to sleep). I'd tell them I'll just put two chairs together. I'm not going away from him. That's not me. If anything, I'll just crawl in bed with him.

Al's grandmother (Regina's mother) Jeanette Fields (right) and her friend Oliver "Mr. Jitterbug" Washington. Jeanette raised nine kids, and she helps considerably in raising her grandchildren.

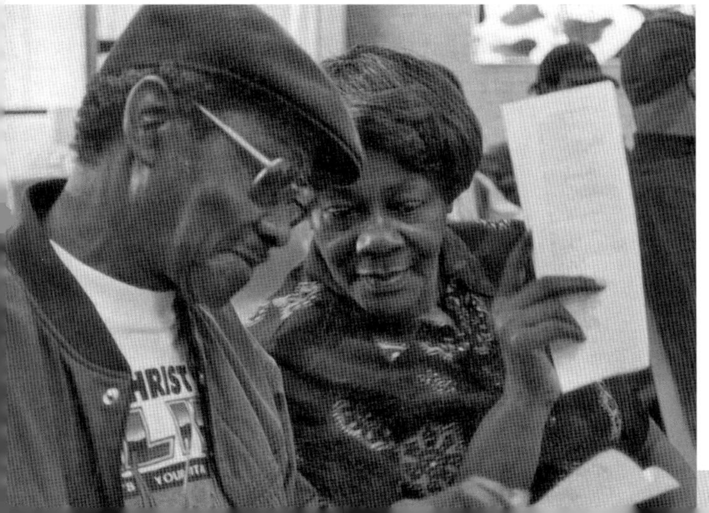

One nurse made me go home one night; I had worked till 11:30 p.m. She said, "Regina, I will be here till 6:00 a.m. I will call you, or I will come get you. Just go home and get some sleep." I said, "No, my baby might wake up, and I won't be here." She said, "Regina, go home, or you may be laying on the other bed beside him. You have been here all night before, you went to work, you need to go home." I said, "That's my baby, my only child!" She kicked me out finally.

I wouldn't wish it on anybody. My son, he was strong with it. I would get depressed.

Yes, I did cry. I didn't cry in front of him because I wanted him to know I could be strong just like him. I cried by myself. It was the loneliest two years I ever went through in my life.

I had my family and stuff. They helped me. My mother, and my sister and them. Some of my brothers. My nephews. And my mother took care of him when I was at work. It would've been harder if she wasn't there.

She just told me, "You have to deal with it. The sadness and all that, you have to look over that and deal with your child." She said the only part that's really going to help him is the part that you be there every day, that he can see your face every day. That helps more than anything. And I was there. Rough and all.

The only time you would see him down is when he had chemo and his counts were down. Anything else, he was in high spirits. When I saw that he could get through it, then I could get through it. Now if he had been depressed, that would have made me depressed. He had a social worker, but I didn't.

When we first went there to the hospital, I forget the family name, their son had just taken his last chemo treatment. He was explaining to the parents and explaining to Al and I the ropes and different things like that. Al made a lot of friends. Some of the friends have passed on, and that kind of bothered him. I told him, "They would want you to keep on going."

He didn't show it, but I think he was scared. Yeah, he was putting up a brave front to protect me.

It just made me stronger. My mother backed me up for hours when I had to work. I didn't get home from work till about twelve. When he got to come home, Al had a C-line in, but he'd clean it. He did everything. They showed me how to do it. I did it for a while, but then he started doing it. He knew it had to be cleaned everyday. Then he had the blood clot in his leg, and I gave the shots a couple weeks. Then he started giving his own shots, because he had to have one in the morning, then one before I came home. He did a lot of things.

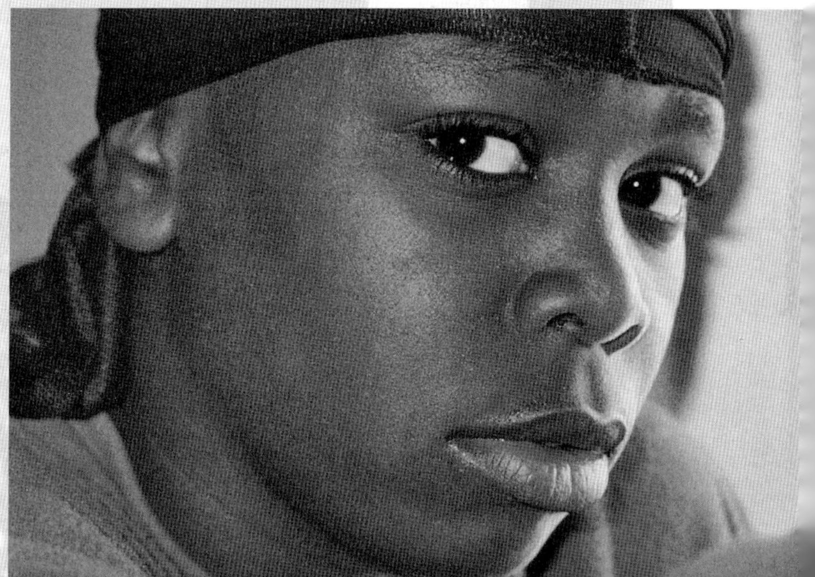

Al looking out the window of his Cincinnati home. He would often look for his mother to return from work, especially on days when he was out of school.

When he got finished with his treatments, they took the all-over x-ray. There must have been a childhood fracture; there was a little piece up here on the x-ray. They kept the C-line in him until three months later. Then they took the C-line out of him, and they said it was all over; come back in six months.

I was watching him for symptoms. When he was sleeping I would run in there and look at him. I get afraid it could come back any minute. That's why I make sure he goes to his clinic

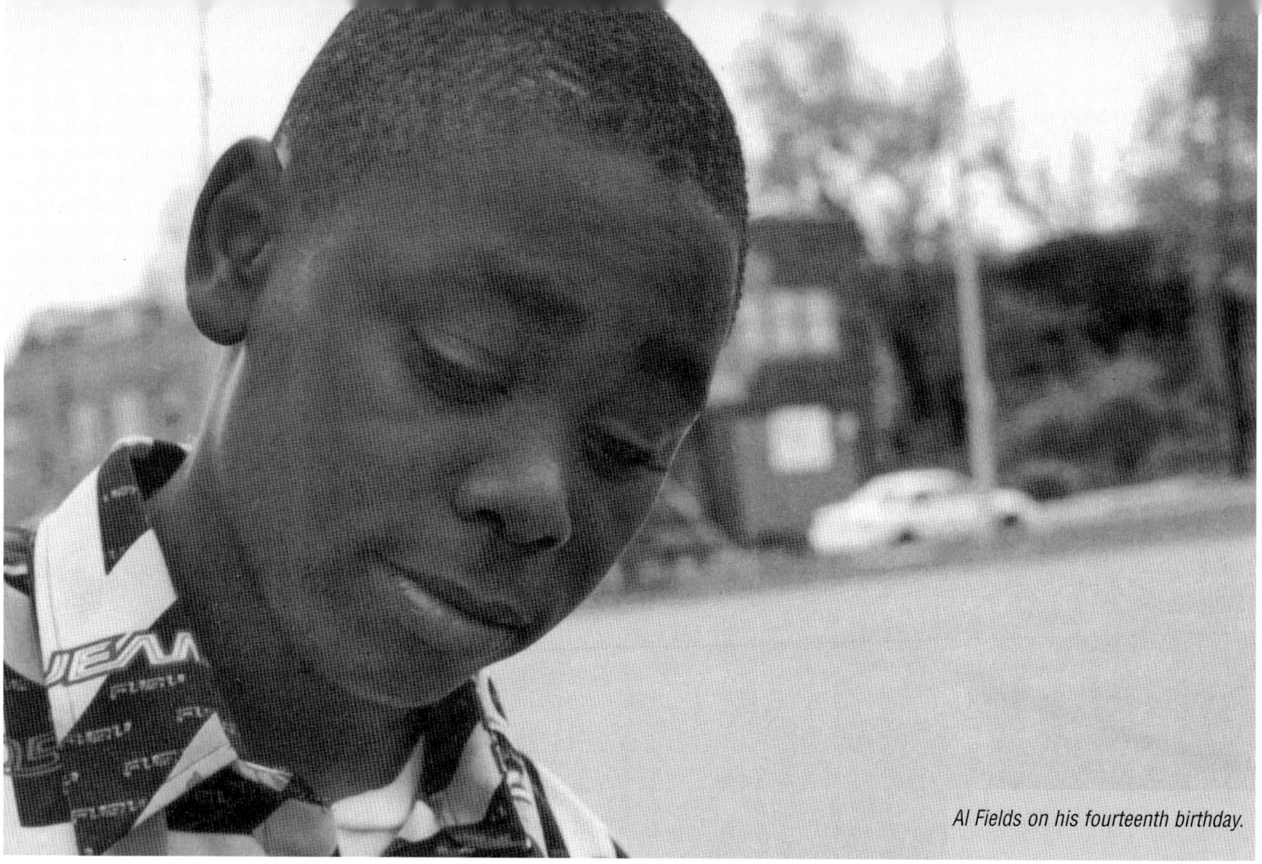
Al Fields on his fourteenth birthday.

appointments, and I go with him, even though he's grown. I go with him. I take off of work and ask questions. The doctor says that sometimes the chemo messes with the muscles in your heart.

They say it's as you get older. Like if he gets older at forty, fifty or sixty years old, he might start having heart problems. That is the reason why they would check it every three months when he was going through chemo.

They do have a behavior problem. They explained to us before they gave him the chemo that he could have problems with behaviors, with attention span. He was bad, hyper and not paying attention in school. They have quick tempers. He did all right in school, but that is when the behaviors started. When the nurse from Children's went to explain to the teachers in the high school, the kids thought that they could catch it by sitting by him. I had the nurse go back and tell them and the teachers that if he was running around and playing and the C-line breaks, what they should do.

With the kids it is just curiosity. They don't know. This was probably the first time they had a schoolmate that had something. It was out in the open. Some people try to hide stuff. I wanted folks to know what to do in case my baby got sick.

The teachers were really nice. They even set up a little room for him if he got too tired. It was a little nap room and water. A kit was there in case something happened.

When Al was sick, we had some wonderful nurses. When he was going to the clinic, we would be there all day, and staff would stop by and say, "Are you all all right?" They would play with the

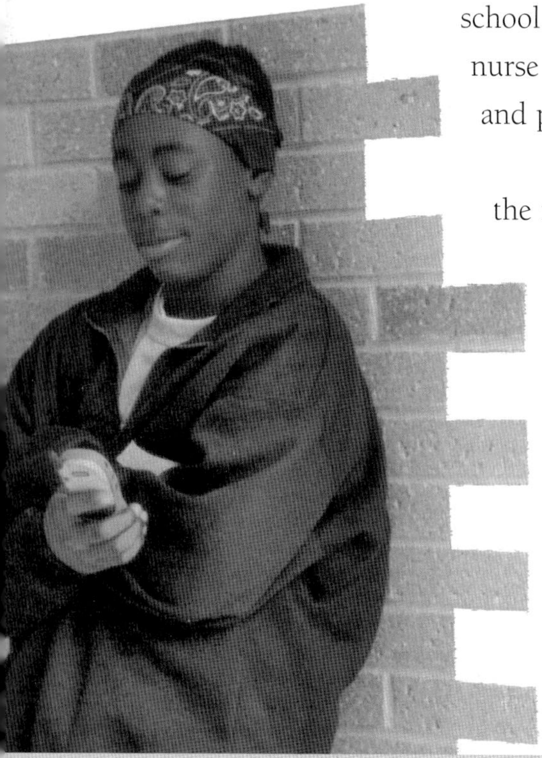
Al looking cool at fourteen.

kids. They would give them a hug, joke, make them smile when they were running around there with their little bald heads. They would compliment them on their caps—the different caps they would have on their heads. Everybody got along. The families got along. You could sit and converse with your family.

I would tell other parents we have the best Children's Hospital. They will take over. We have the best doctors over there for kids with cancer. Trust them. They are good at explaining things to you. They are good, they really are.

That part, going for treatment, is over. It is the part that is out there that is scary. Dealing with him out on the street is different than dealing with him ill. It is rough out there for a young man out on the street.

Yeah, he takes health for granted sometimes. He grew up fast. He did. He grew up before he should have been grown because he had to go through that. Now, he can't sit still.

He does feel more for other kids than most teenagers. He always tries to be somebody's boss. He's a daddy figure. To his little cousin, he's the daddy figure. He's supposed to mind him. They listen.

Al's been a handful since he was born. A handful. I'm Virgo and he's Taurus; we're both bullheaded. We're going to get our point across. He likes to fight. (Teachers would report) "'He did this and he did that," and then he come along and say he didn't do it. Which he did do it. Little kid stuff. Being bad. Original bad. But he don't steal. He don't do drugs. He doesn't even drink. He's just an ornery, ordinary boy. He's got a sensitive side to him. And he likes his sports. As long as you let him do his sports, he's happy.

When you are doing it by yourself, it is hard to do anything. All I did was do it. You will do anything for a child that is sick. Now that I have been through this with Al, I know how other parents feel. I can say, "I know how you feel, and these are the steps that I took. Put it in the hands of the Lord." That's what I did. God can look over my child when I can't.

Sometimes I think, "Was my baby really sick?" 'Cause he didn't go through none of that. After two years they said it was gone. I was like, "Was you for real?"

He blocks some out. It will never leave him, but he kind of blocks it. He wants to be like a normal person, "I'm like anybody else."

Now, it's girls, girls, girls. He is always with girls. My phone rings off the hook with girls. He has so much he

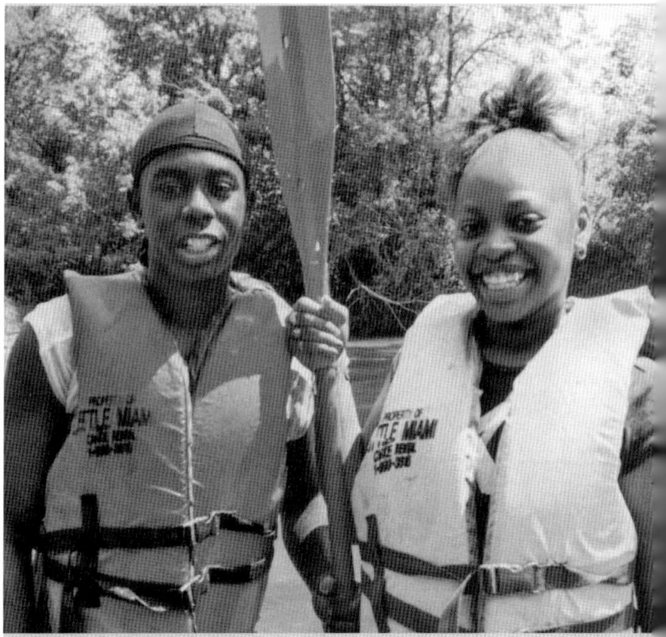

Al and his cousin Jené on a canoeing trip north of Cincinnati.

Al at seventeen years old.

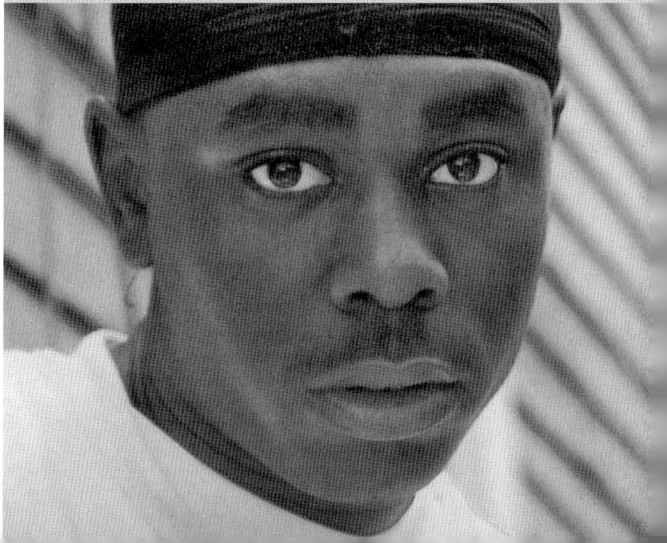

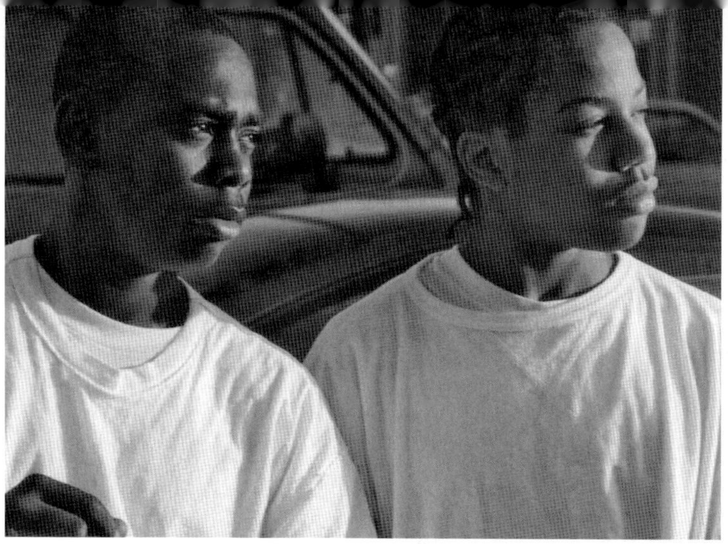

Al and his cousin Khalid, a.k.a. Nook.

wants to do. You never know about Alex. One time he wants to do this; the next time he wants to do that. He was into basketball in the film. Then he went to rap. You never know about that boy.

Sometimes he get tired of being asked about it. Ask Steve and Julia. When they were interviewing him, he'd want them to go away.

He was in the hospital when the movie first started and he first got sick. They got this social worker who set up the home schooling. She asked me, "Would you like to be in a documentary?" I said, "You've got to ask him." He said, "Yeah."

Sometimes Julia and Steve would get there so early in the morning that he was a little grumpy. "No, no more cameras, Mommy. No more cameras." Sometimes I could just look and they knew to cool it down. Let me tell you, it took them a whole year to get an interview with me. I'd say, "I don't feel like it tonight. I don't feel like it today." It was a whole year. They cornered me at the hospital.

Oh, and my baby just loves pictures. He thinks he's a star already. You should have seen him with the interviews when we were in Texas. He pushed me back and said, "Mama, let me do the talking." That was at the Lance Armstrong Foundation. That was really nice. They still call and send us letters and stuff. Even nurses would send him cards and stuff. I tell him, "Oh, you must have been a good baby."

Julia and Steve are good friends too. Julia's daughter had the same kind of cancer Al had. They are good people. They would come get him for his birthday. His eighteenth birthday, every birthday since they met him, they would take him out for his birthday. They would come and get him and take him home with them. They rode bikes and motorcycles. They took him to see the animals.

I told them they could adopt him. I said, "If I'm gone, I'll leave him to you." They were good with him. Him and Steve are just like this. Steve is a lovely person. Julia is all right. Steve is a sweet, sensitive guy. Julia is like, "Come on Regina; come on Regina." Steve is like, "Julia, let Regina think about it." I'd be sitting there cracking up about it.

Every story that is in the movie, I'll be boo-hooing like I don't know what. Very sad, but very true. They need to show it. It affects everybody whether you are rich, poor, black, white, green or yellow. It isn't a race disease.

Al Fields remains cancer-free. He hopes to attend college near home.

Dr. Huang, he's a cool doctor. He will tell me if he thinks something's wrong and I shouldn't do it. But if it's something he thinks is okay and he know it's safe for me, he will let me do it. Like I was supposed to go to Colorado (to a camp), and I couldn't go because my counts was low, but he was going to let me go. I had to get my chemo before I could go to Colorado; he tried to give me stuff to get my counts up, so I could go to Colorado, but I just couldn't go because my counts was too low.

Sue (Sealock) and Nikki (Schaefer), they my favorite nurses. Sue, she just funny, and she's a good nurse too. She like taking care of her kids in the clinic. She take care of her kids in the clinic like they were really her kids.

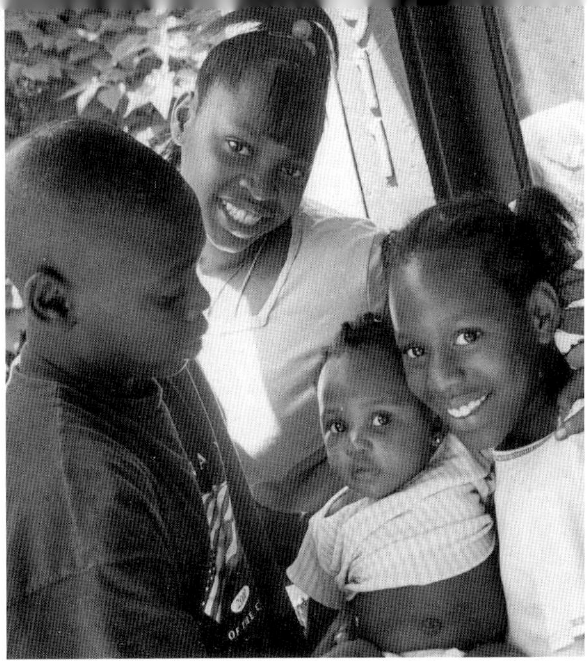

Al and his cousins on the porch of his grandmother's house.

When my mom knew I was getting hot, and I couldn't breathe, and I was coughing a lot, she took me to the hospital. And the doctors in the emergency kept coming in and out, looking at my chest. My mom was sad, she kind of knew what it was. She had a feeling. But then they took me up and gave me a CAT scan, and they said what it was. I started crying. That was the scariest moment. There was this one Chinese lady, I can't remember her name. They said I was going to die or I was going to live, and I had to fight it.

I thought my mama was having a seizure when the doctor told me, this one doctor with glasses. When he told me I was looking just like (makes an expression showing shock). I'm looking at my mama just making sure she hadn't hit her head, the way she was acting. For real, 'cause she was. I thought she was losing it. 'Cause he blurted it out. "Alex, I have a diagnosis of cancer, and in the area of the top of his chest there is a mass." My mama was flipping out, pushing the bed, about to tip me over.

When she started flipping out, I knew it was up to me, because she was looking bad. Crying. Falling over the place. I was only eleven; I was scared to death, but I was holding it in. I didn't cry, cry, cry because the Chinese lady told me I would be okay. But I wanted to smack the dude with the glasses.

Then after all of the doctors left, my mama just told me to pray in the bed; then I started praying. She told me I had to get on my knees to pray, but I can still pray in the bed while I'm laying down.

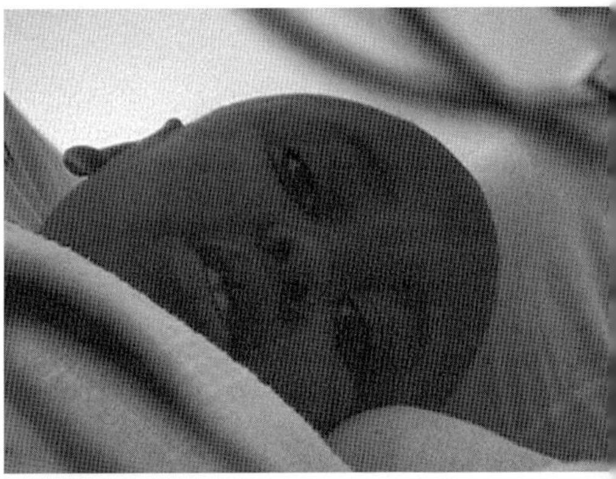

Alex "Al" Fields shortly after his diagnosis of non-Hodgkin's lymphoma.

Then I didn't talk to nobody. I didn't even talk to my cousins. They would come see me, and I would be asleep or whatever or acting like I was asleep. To tell you the truth, I was in the hospital so long, I thought I was in there for the whole summer. I don't know how many weeks I was in there. I know I wasn't eating that food. That food was nasty.

I'm the only person that my mom's got. Besides her mom and her brothers and stuff. She felt that she ain't want to lose her child 'cause I'm the only child. That just made me stay strong.

She causes me lots of stress. But she's good. She helped me. She

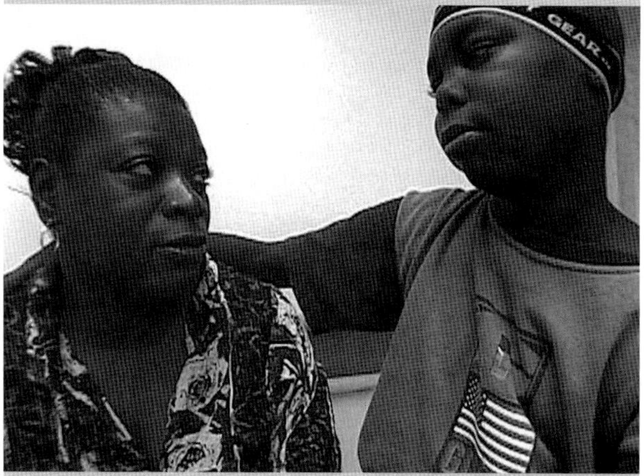

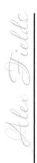

Al and his mother, Regina, size each other up between rounds of verbal sparring.

basically was the only one who tried to make me feel better. Most of the time, her and my grandma. She was considerate, helpful, you can tell she was sad, but she didn't let me know she was sad. But when I was sad, she was sad, and I didn't want to let her know I was sad either. I could tell she was scared.

I started getting more mature. I started acting less, and I just started being myself. A new person that's me, clean and healthy.

I never thought about (dying). I tried to keep it from my head and tried to live normal like I usually did. The more you think about it, the more you worry about it. Basically, I just chilled. The only thing that was so hard on me was I had to learn not to worry about what other people think at school, because I didn't even want to go to school. The year I left school I had a teacher, her name was Ms. Miller. She had cancer. But then when I got it, and came back to school, she died. Then we had to make letters to our parents and all of that.

Even though I looked different, I knew I wasn't different. I was the same old person. I lost hair. I was skinnier and everything. They didn't make fun of me. But I was getting looked at.

I ain't changed. I have always been strong. It made my mama stronger and me wiser. Before I started coming to the clinic, I didn't know all about the shots and all that. While my mama was learning, she didn't know I was learning, because I was always with a cover up over my head or keeping quiet. But I listened to what she was doing, and I watched. Then I started learning about different parts on the body, different types of cancer, and stuff like that.

Last year in school we had a quiz about leukemia, and I got my test right, and the teacher asked me how I knew all the symptoms and all that about people with cancer and how they feel. I said, "I don't know." We don't need to get all into that. I just know more about it now.

I learned how to treat life. You ain't always going to be here tomorrow, so live life like you can today.

What kind of advice would I give other kids? Keep their head up and just don't worry about it; just go with the flow. But never get depressed or never get real, real sick, 'cause that will just make you sicker. Go out and don't think about it. And if you in the hospital, don't try to sleep the day over, try to have some fun. 'Cause if you sleep it over, that will make you get depressed.

I would tell them that it is going to be okay. Try to be strong. And if you do pass, then you'll be with the Lord. Either way you go, you still got it good. That's it. This is all I got to say to all the kids out there, just keep your head up, it's going to be all right.

Filmmakers' Journal

Julia: Regina is one of the most direct people I know. She just tells it as it is. She's a woman of few words, but each one counts. Her opinions are clear and strong, and she lets you know them. I think this is one way she's managed to raise a firecracker of a kid like Al, and all his cousins too. Regina has been the primary parent figure for some of Al's cousins. The Fields family is really tight. They value family and they stick together, even if they don't always get along. A lot of the credit for the strong family has to go to Regina's mother, who raised nine kids. Regina learned a lot from her mom about how to be a strong parent.

Steven: When we first started filming them, Al was the most withdrawn young man. He was so quiet and always hiding under a sheet. I wondered if we had picked the wrong family or if maybe this kid wasn't ever going to come out of his shell. Boy, was I wrong. Pretty soon Al had us and his mother chasing him all over the hospital.

When we first met him, he was a still a short little kid. This was back in the late 1990s, and the big news in recent years had been the Clinton sex scandals. So there we are following Al around, and Regina's walking with us too, and one day she says, "Al, they're following you around 'cuz they think you're Bill Clinton's secret son." We all laughed, and for the rest of the day, Regina was repeating it everywhere we went, stage whispering "That's Clinton's son!" We couldn't stop laughing, even though we were getting some strange looks.

Julia: Al had a growth spurt pretty quick. It seemed like he grew four or five inches in one year. Soon he was a really outgoing, energetic twelve-year-old. His favorite nurse was Nikki—Nicole Schaefer. He loved Nikki and she adored Al and had the ability to keep him in line. But who really kept him in line was Regina. She had such an arsenal, such a tool kit to do the job. She could switch on a dime from making him laugh and giving him such warm comfort to scolding him and giving him that tough love.

There was one time when Al was giving his mom a lot of lip. They were in the hospital, and Regina had to go. Al started complaining that she never spent enough time with him. Which is crazy, because she did. But he's just a kid, and he didn't want his mom to go. He's giving her all this grief, and he's got his attitude up. He starts saying something like, "Well, if you don't want to be here, then go." And he just starts repeating "Bye. Bye." Regina tries talking to him, but he's just in her face. So she finally says, "Okay. Bye." And she gets up, gets her purse, and leaves. It shocked him. He got really quiet after that. A little while later, he asked us, "She left?" He seemed to get three years younger in one moment.

That kind of moment says a lot about the really tricky balance a parent has to have with a kid who has cancer. We saw this in all the families. You so want to spoil your kid, because they are suffering so much. But you can't. Like Scott Lougheed said, if you do spoil them, you could have a monster on your hands before you know it. Regina accused the nurses and us of spoiling Al: "You all spoil him and then send him home to me." She was right too.

Steven: Cincinnati went through some real upheaval while we were filming. There was a series of incidents where young, unarmed African American men were killed by Cincinnati police officers. When a young man named Timothy Thomas was shot in an alley by a cop he was running from, it sparked days of rioting and almost a state of martial law in Cincinnati. It was huge news here, and it made national news too. And here's young Al, just at that critical age of thirteen or fourteen, where he's starting to wander the streets during the daytime, and he lives in a really hard hit neighborhood. We were worried about him—about the gang influences in his neighborhood, about the police harassing him, about his own occasional salty attitude getting the best of him at the wrong moment.

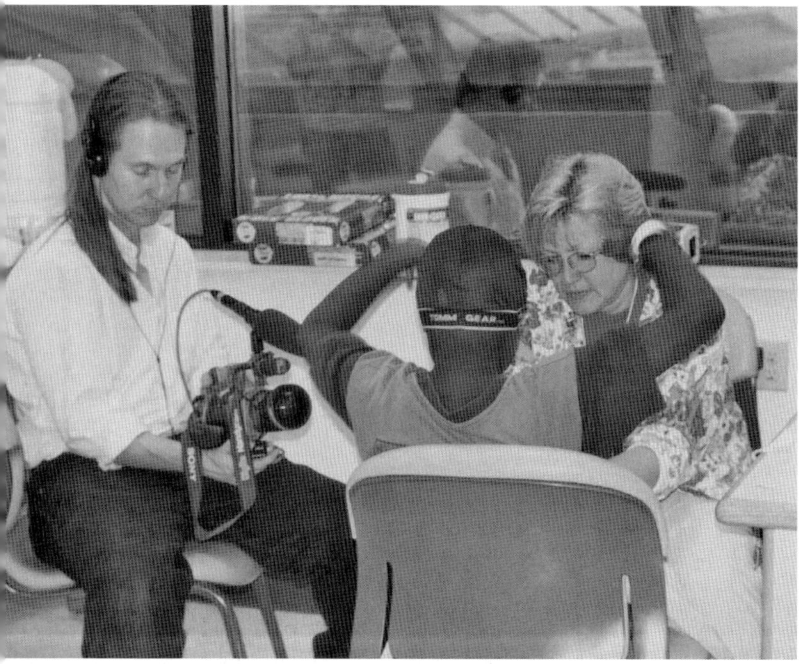

Steve films Alex in the early days, as his nurse checks his C-line.

He has a temper, and it flares sometimes. We talked to him about it. It turns out Regina and the other adults in the family had really talked to all the kids about how you talk to cops, how you don't run from them, how you avoid trouble on the streets. But it was a scary time. A few years later, Regina summed up the dangers of cancer and the dangers Al faces in life when she said, "I don't worry about him going back to the doctor's office. I worry about him running the streets. The streets are more dangerous than the doctor's office."

Julia: Al has turned into a pretty wonderful young man. He's very thoughtful, really kind.

Steven: He went to Sundance, even though Regina had to stay home. We're grateful to him and the Moones for going out there even though we had already left. Beth Moone said that Al was just so thoughtful, and he was always looking out for Beth's mother, Jen's grandma, always helping her get through the snow banks and being considerate of her.

Julia: I'm really glad Al and Jen got to hang out. I wish we could have been there for that. I still want to see them and Jen's sister Natalie play some basketball together.

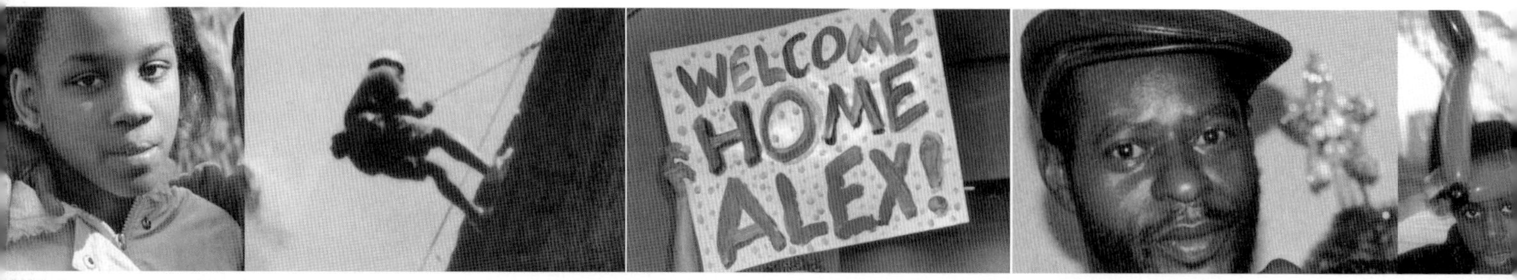

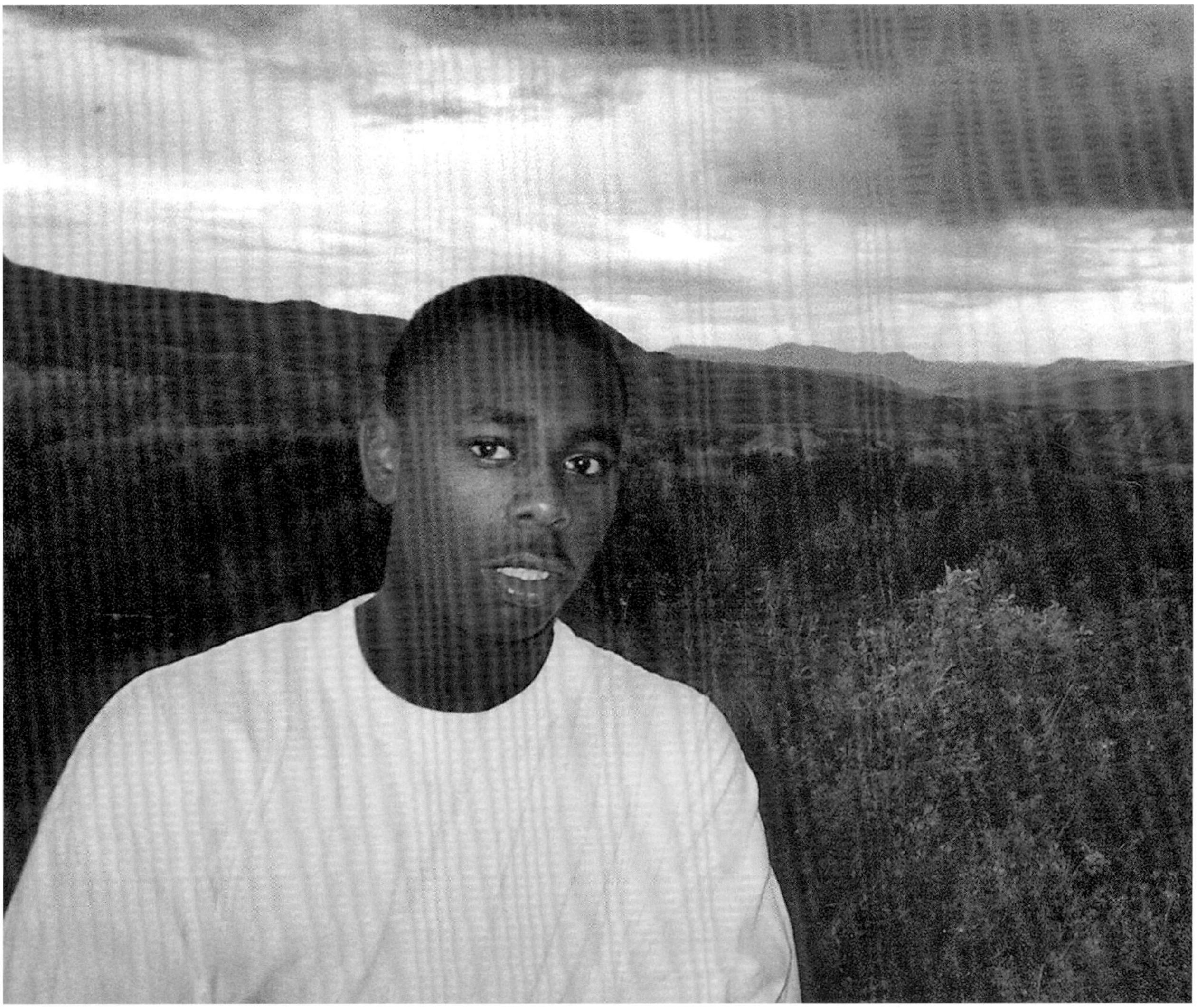

Alex finally makes it to camp in Colorado. In the film, Alex goes from excited to disappointed when he learns he can't go to camp because his blood counts are too low. Four years later, Alex finally went to Colorado, attending First Descents, a kayaking camp for young adult survivors of childhood cancer.

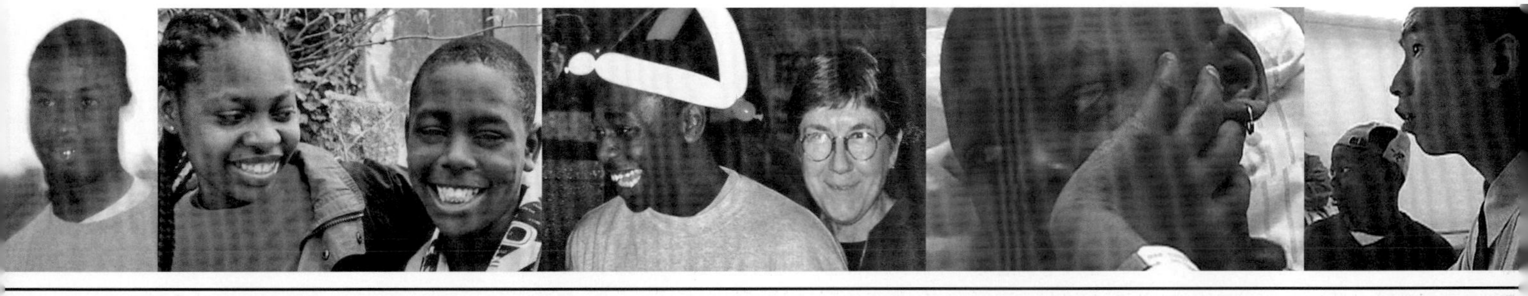

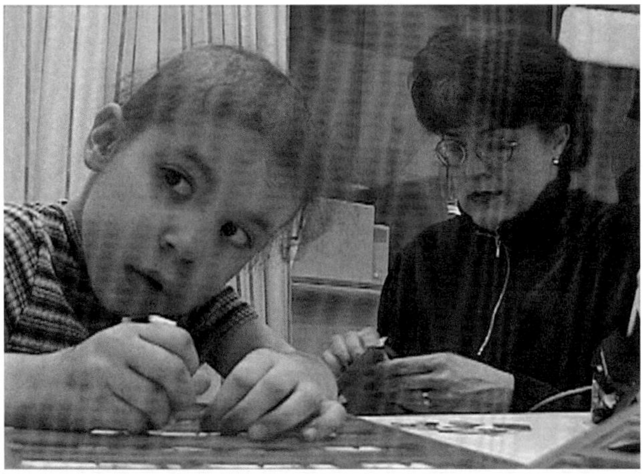

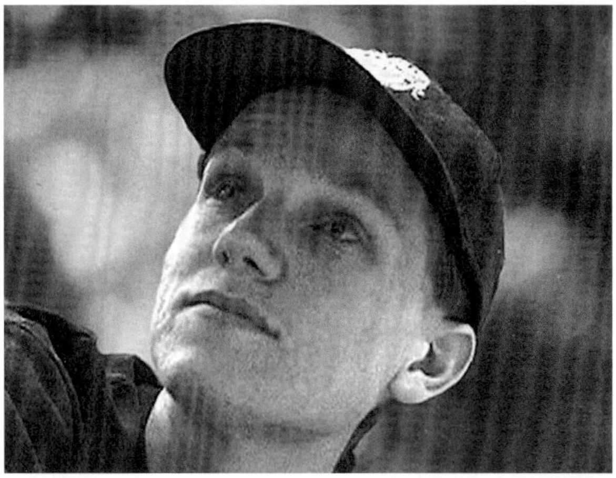

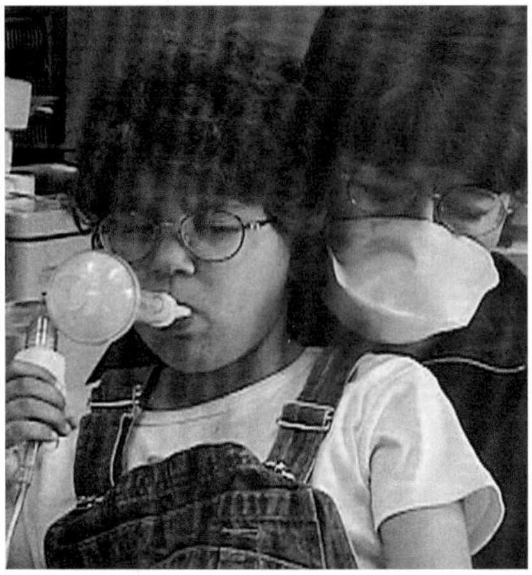

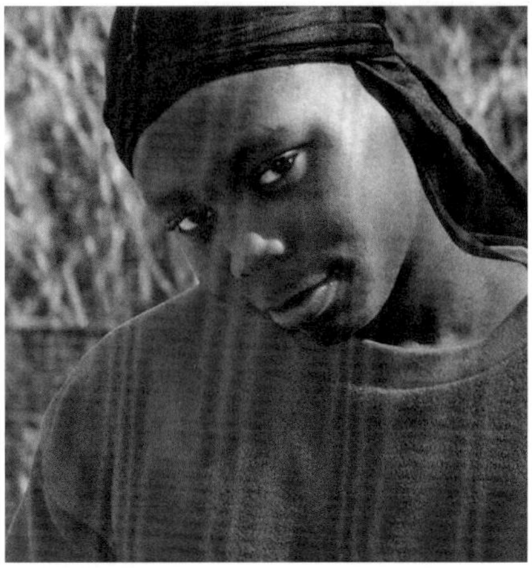

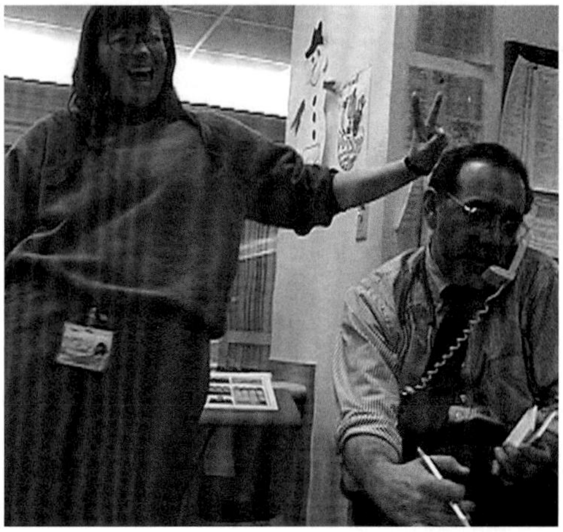

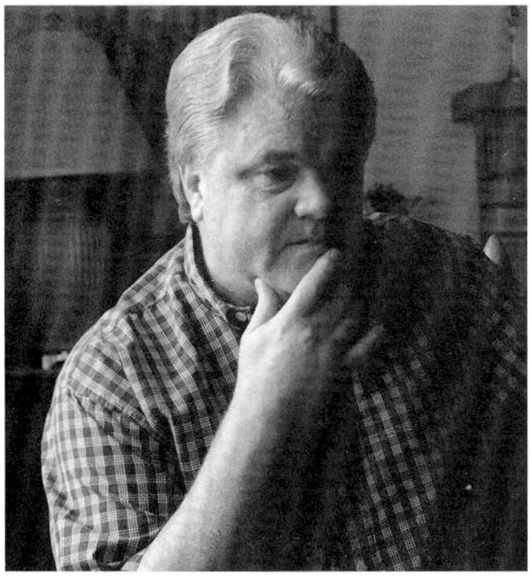

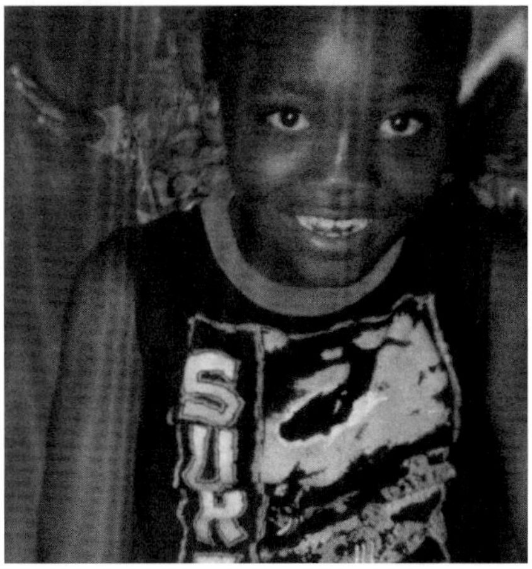

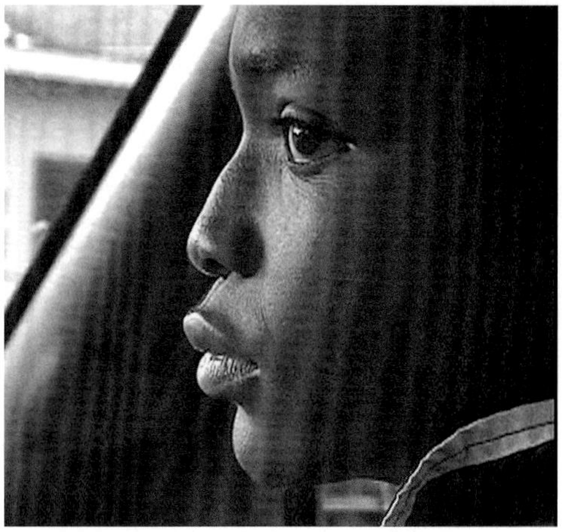

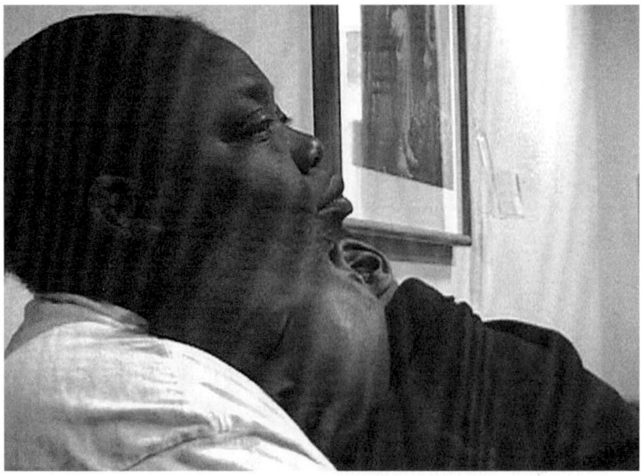

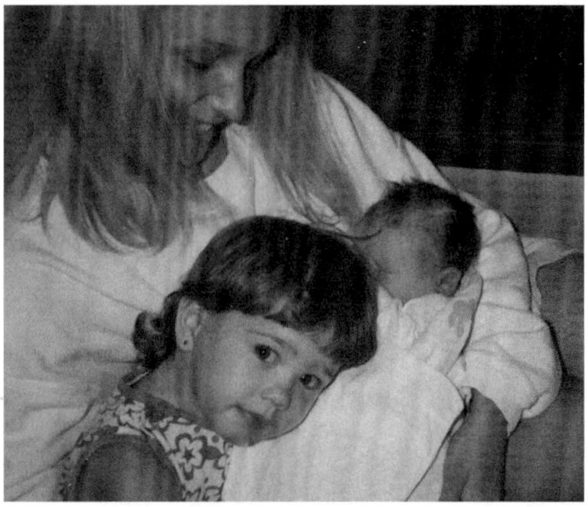

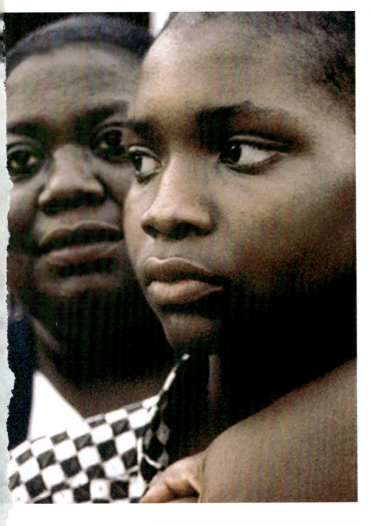

“Odds are for people with no faith. I don’t run out of faith. Medically, we have no options; spiritually, we have plenty.”
—Marietha Woods.

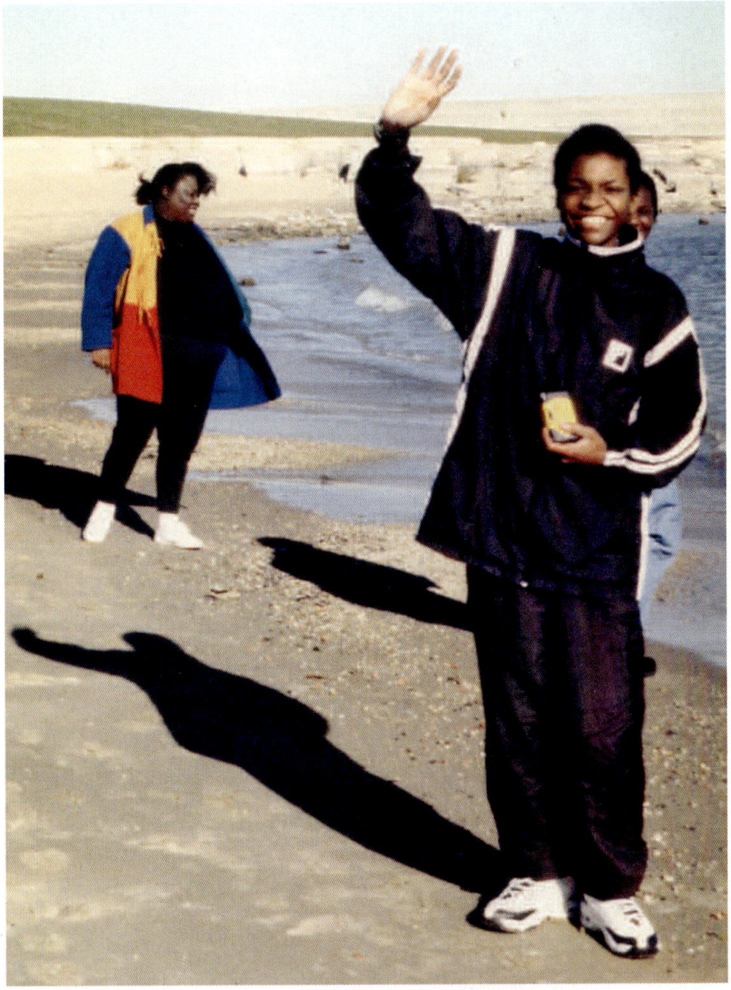

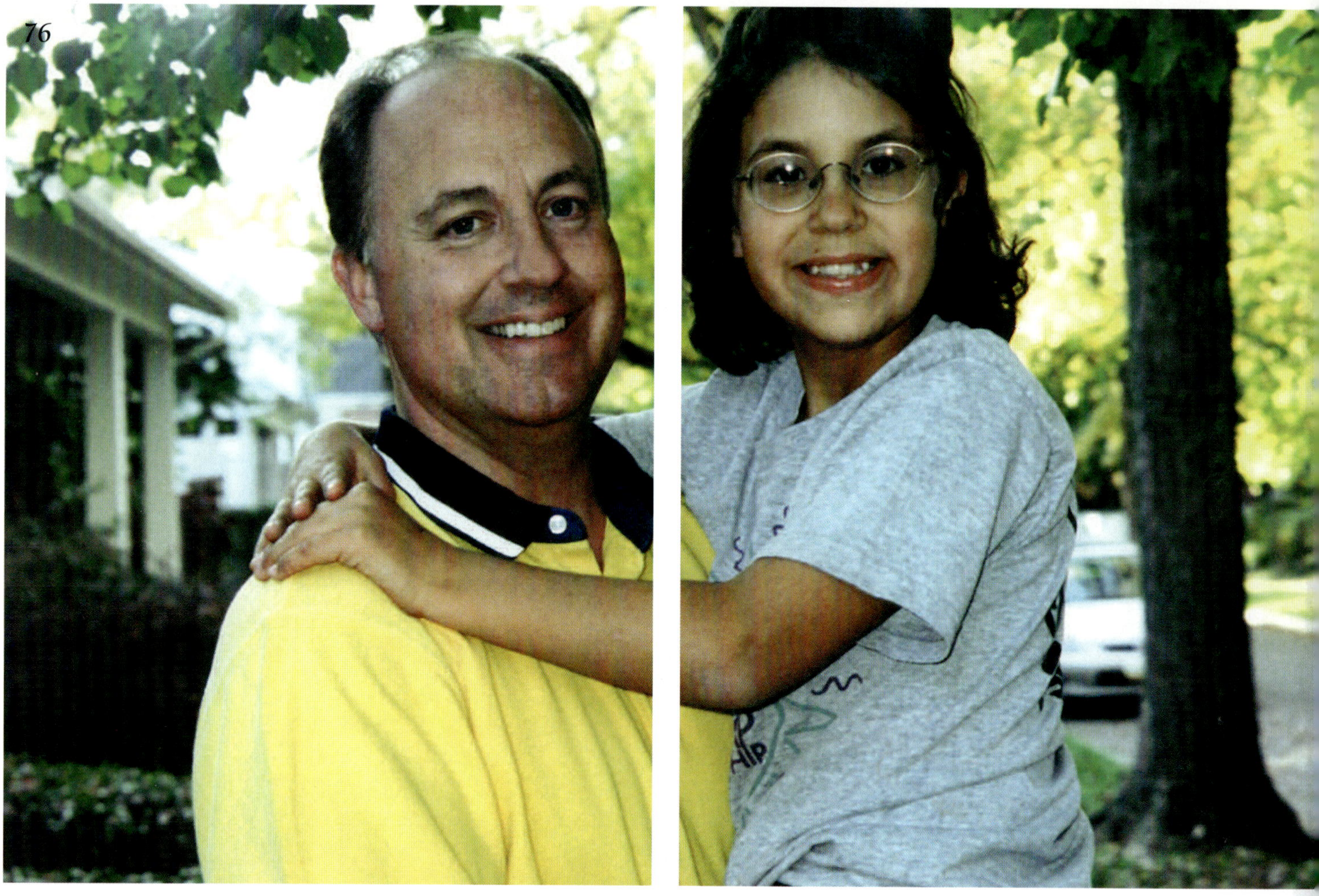

"I feel like I'm just more conscious of what's really important. The things I thought were important, they mean nothing."—Beth Moone

"I missed silly things. I'd go to Starbucks and see women dressed up in suits, and think, 'Gosh, that used to be me. And now I have sweats on. I don't wear make up.' It's a different me. Before I was a half-time mom. Now I'm a full-strength mom."

—Beth Moone

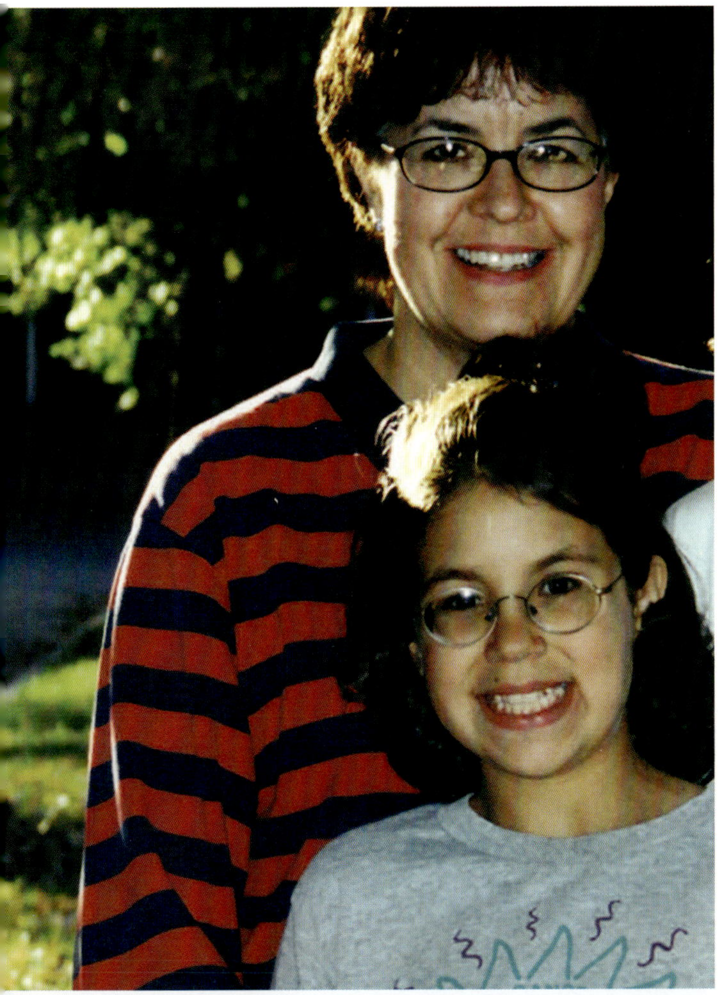

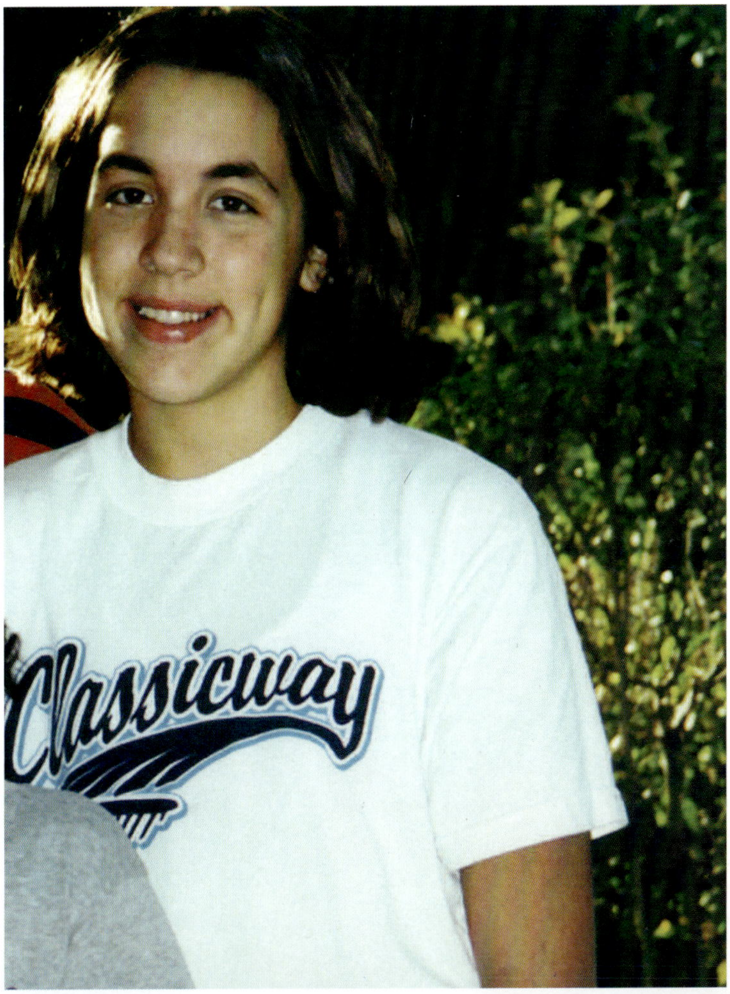

"Don't take anything for granted. Don't let a day go by where you don't hug your kids and tell them you love them. Tell them how special they are."
—Judy Lougheed

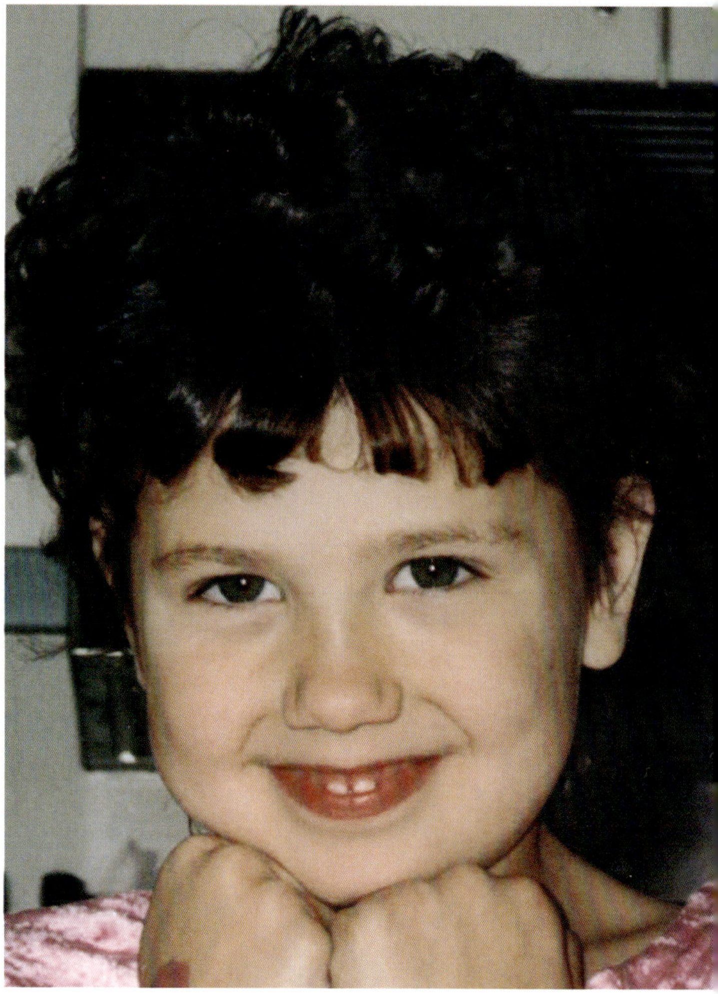

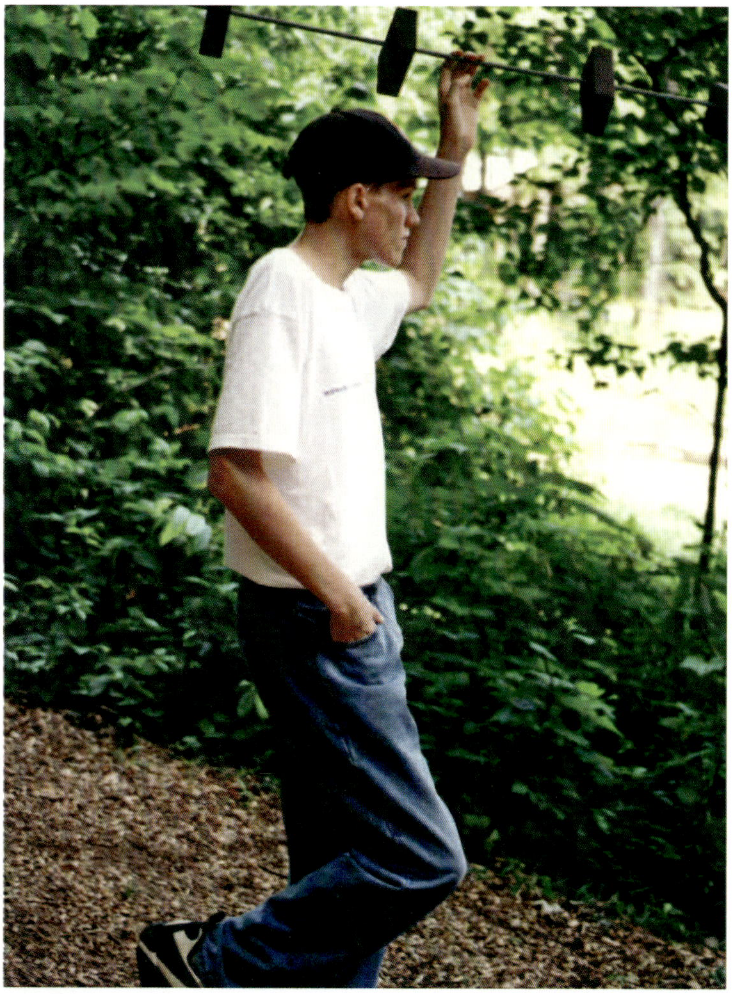

"This is the way I was from day one with this illness: Be positive. Don't dwell on things. Go forward."
—Debbie Kenner

"To me, children that have cancer are so beyond their age group. They've had to grow up real quick. Life to them—they don't take life for granted like teenagers do. It's very important to them. They want to live it."
—Debbie Kenner

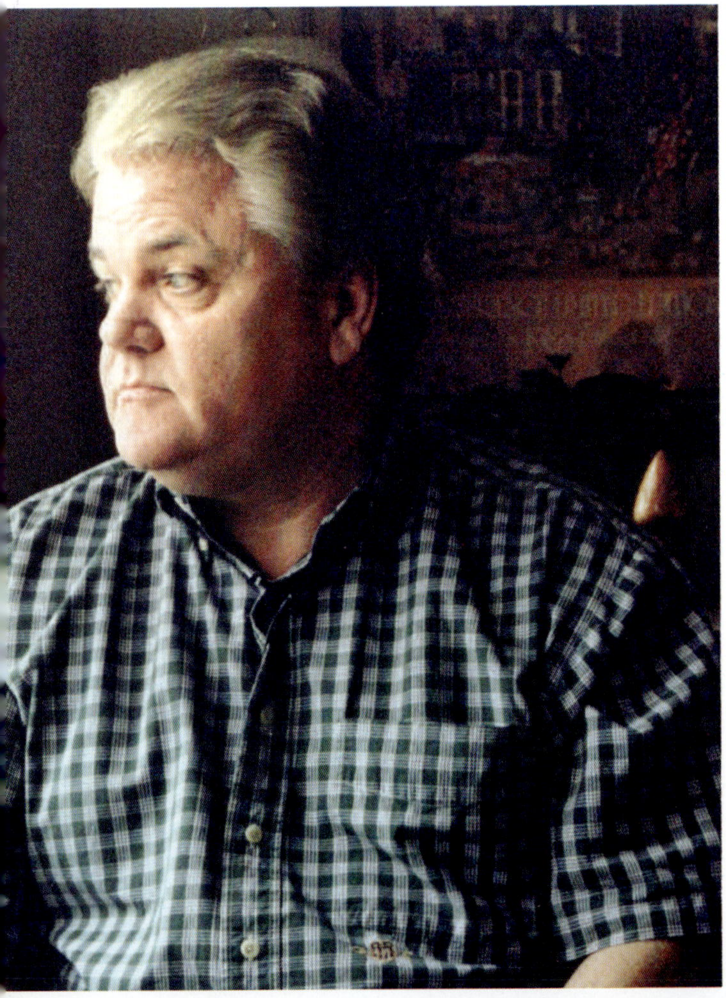

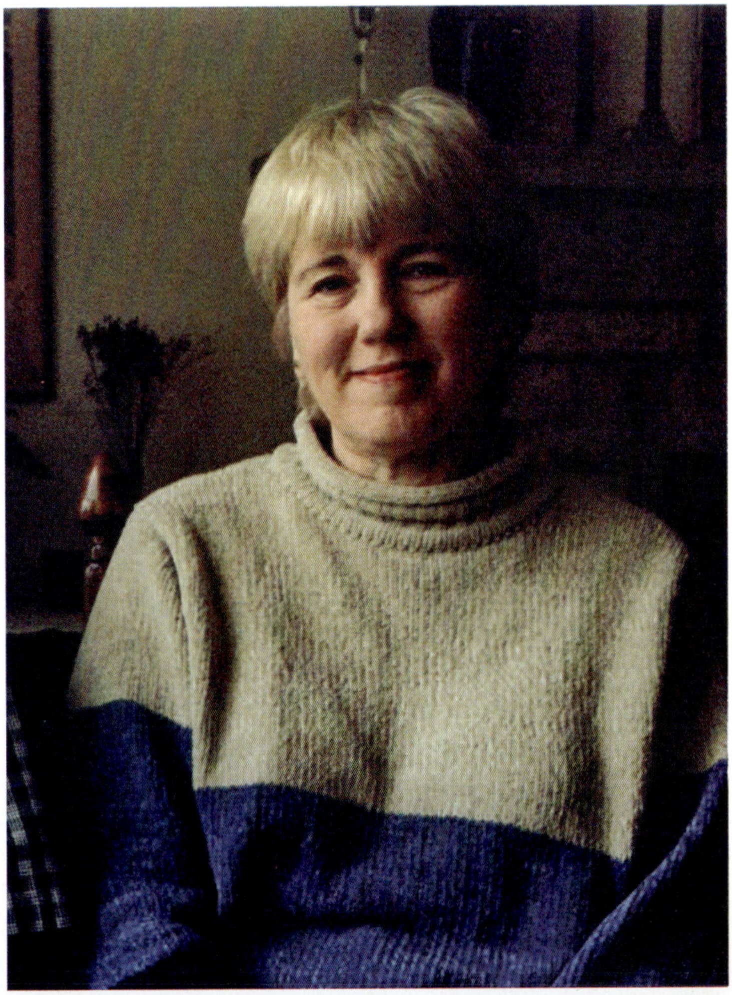

"What do I wish I knew on that day? How hard it was going to be."
—Scott Lougheed

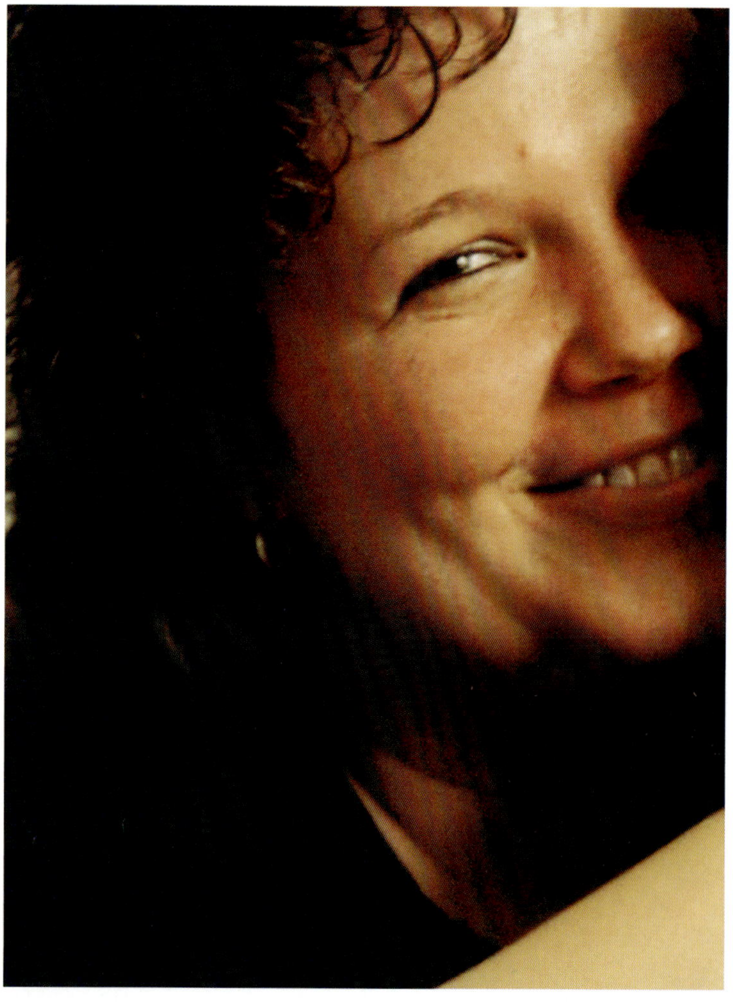

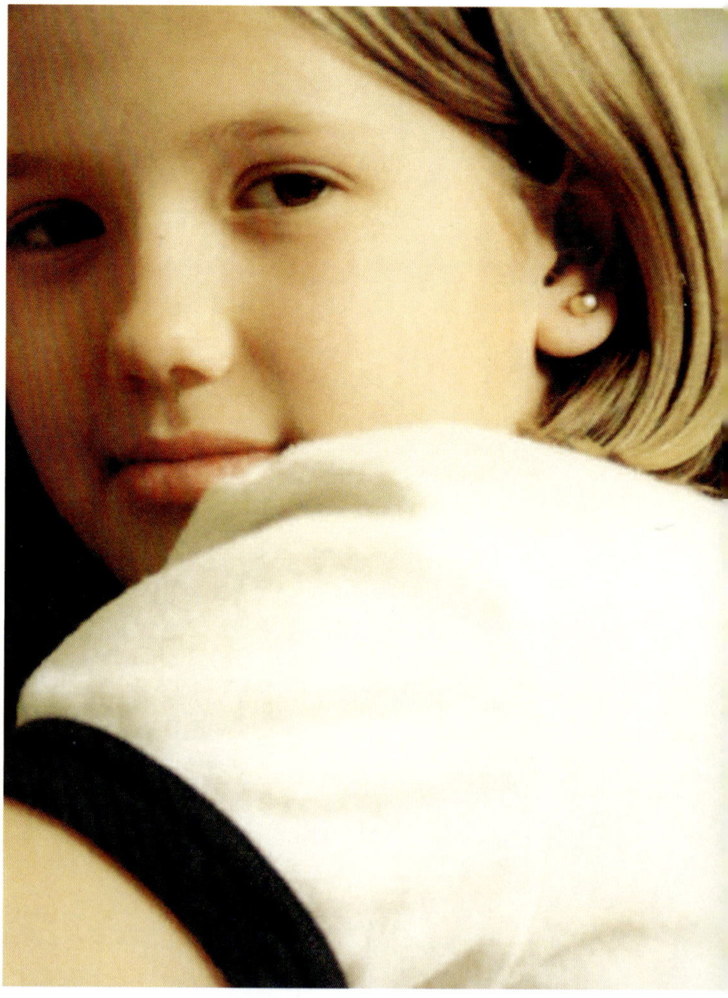

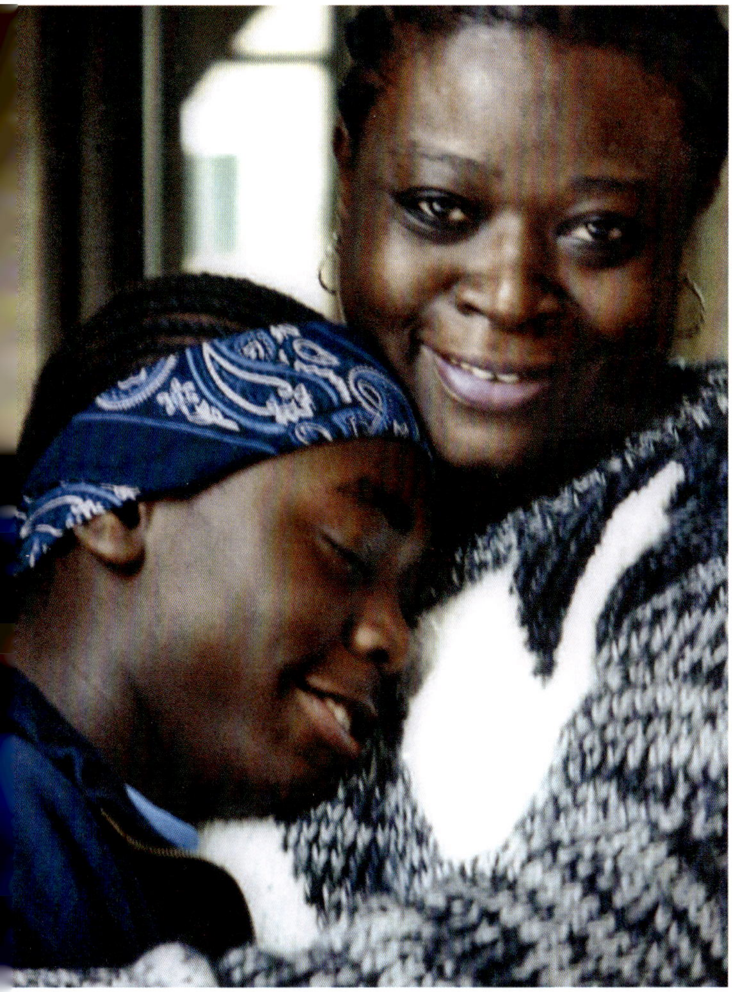

"They tried to give me this room away from him (to sleep). I'd tell them I'll just put two chairs together. I'm not going away from him. That's not me."
—Regina Fields

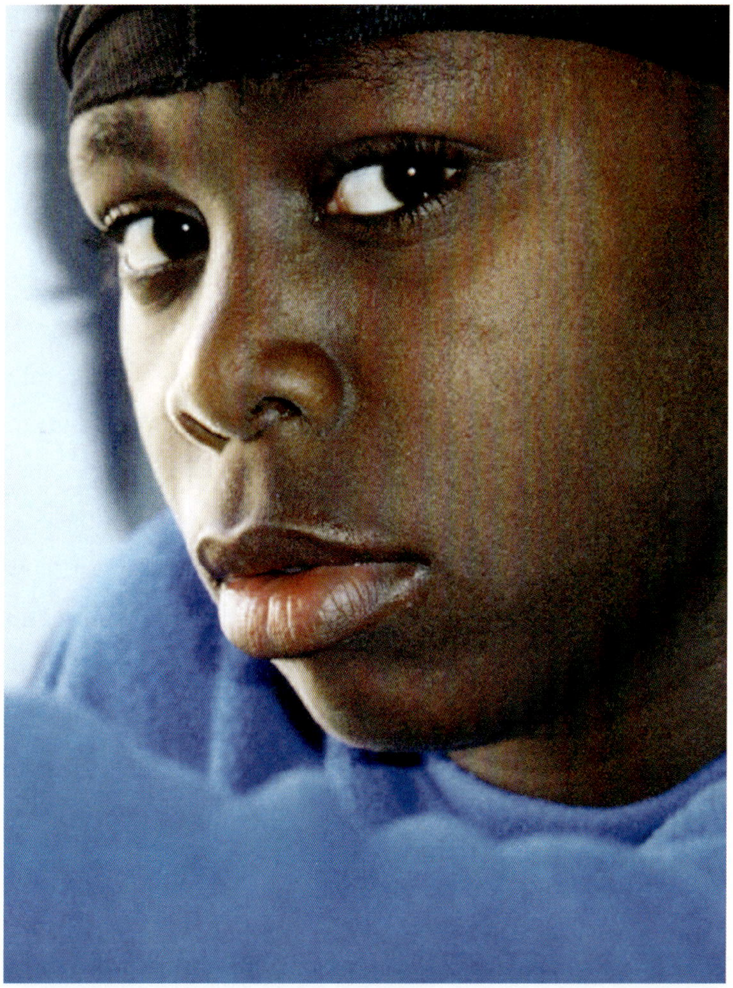

Chapter 6

Robert ARCECI

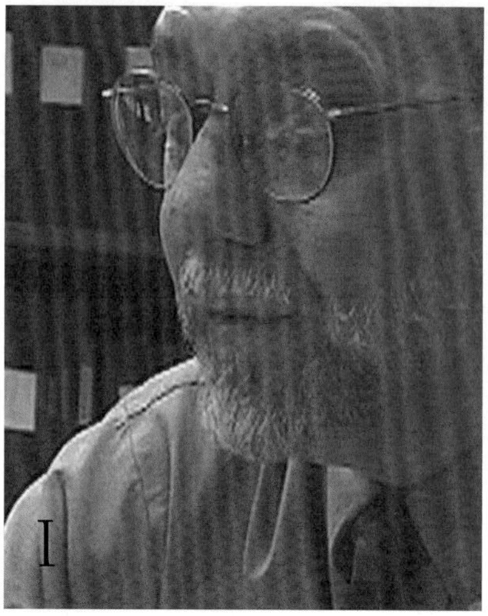

robertARCECI, M.D., Ph.D

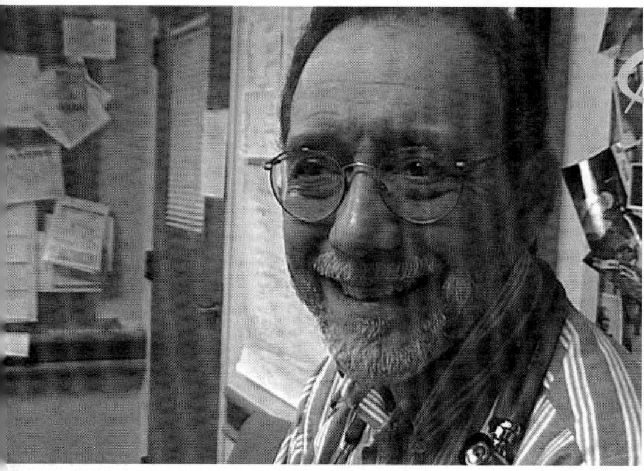

Dr. Arceci was head of Cincinnati Children's Hospital Medical Center Hematology/Oncology Division when he saw "Personal Belongings," a biographical documentary by Steven Bognar, that aired on public television as part of the "P.O.V." documentary series. He was sufficiently impressed to contact Bognar and his partner Julia Reichert to invite them to come to make a movie about some of his patients and their parents. He is now the King Fahd Professor and Director of Pediatric Oncology at Johns Hopkins University School of Medicine.

I had wanted to make a movie about childhood cancer from the point of view of the patients' families and caretakers for quite a long time. When I went to Ohio I had seen Steven's documentary. I was so impressed.

Hoop Dreams, I was very impressed by that documentary. I felt that that documentary was telling it honestly and there were enormous things to be learned from it. I may have mentioned it several times that a movie in the spirit of *Hoop Dreams* would capture what I had been thinking of for so many years. This has been something I wanted to see for twenty years. This was not a fly-by-night interest.

It was then when Julia, Steve and I talked and got things going. I always said, from the beginning, that this would be their movie, and hoped that they would keep it in the spirit of educational focus and representation of these players in this story—to be upfront.

I think early on it was difficult for many people to come to grips with being recorded. For me, it probably lasted for a millisecond of living by the rule of not saying something (for the camera) that I wouldn't say for another person. I don't care who's hearing it or who's recording. This was our work. This is what the movie was about. There was absolutely no reason for anyone to feel that they should portray anything other than their honest appraisal or honest feelings. From my perspective, I forgot that there was a camera or a microphone there. Julia and Steve were exquisitely skilled at making themselves invisible. They are professional and sensitive people. That professional skill is transmitted in the utmost, careful way.

They have used me quite frequently to review excerpts, to discuss content, to discuss things outside the film that would have impact, what to include. I also, very early on, made sure that they had lists of people not associated with the film, colleagues of mine that I thought would be insightful and helpful. I am very much encouraged that they took me up on this, that they would have other people give them input into the field.

I do remember one extraordinary evening in Greenwich Village, when my wife and I and my two sons went to New York City. We got together with Steve and Julia in a little tiny apartment. They were doing some of the editing. They asked if I would mind looking at an excerpt that might or might not be in the film. Of course, this was early on. They wanted to get a feel if this was too much or okay for the film. They were extraordinarily sensitive to the human side of these issues. They wanted to make sure they were accurate and honest, but also that this was not being done for shock value.

At the time, my wife was a little concerned that this might be tough for the kids to see. They were teenagers. We sat there and watched it. It was a scene where I was telling a mother that her son had a malignancy that was not going to be curable and that we should start to plan for his death. At the end of that sequence they asked our children what they thought. Fascinatingly they both independently said, "You know, we actually quite never appreciated what he did for work." It was a very powerful moment. It was moments like that that really stuck in my mind as we went through and edited, scenes they thought might have made a place or a person look less glamorous or less good. Yet the educational content of those scenes was so extraordinary; often we would come down on the side of sensitive honesty.

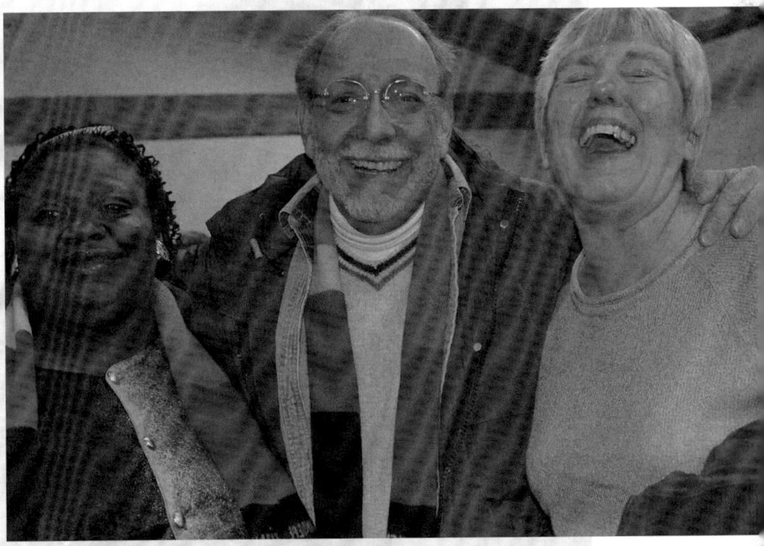

Marietha Woods, Dr. Arceci and Debbie Kenner, at the 2006 Sundance Film Festival.

The movie contains a scene of a meeting where the staff confronts the fact that they have run out of ways to fight Alex Lougheed's cancer and that she will not survive.

Dr. Arceci reads a passage from The Plague *by Albert Camus that concludes, "Until my dying day, I shall refuse to love a scheme of things in which children are put to torture."*

I often will bring literature to the table. There are people out there, one of them is

Albert Camus, who think deeply about these issues of life and death. I have been reading *The Plague* probably since I was about sixteen years old.

I must say that in all the years that I had practiced, that (Alexandra's) situation had ranked in the top in terms of its true horror to true tragedy. It was devastating, of course, for the child. It was just horrific for the family.

I could sense that the house staff and nursing staff were having a difficult time coping with what to do. These are circumstances where it's not about medicine anymore. It's about trying to understand transitions and understand meaning in some personal way. It is just extraordinary to watch this happen. We could have gone over the electrolytes, the chest x-ray, the blood counts, the pain management and then make rounds. But there was an elephant in the room and we had to deal with it straight on. That elephant was what was happening and what we could do very little about.

There just happened to be an extraordinary scene of a dying child in *The Plague*. That scene in my mind has always been quite remarkable because it has all of us in it. We have all of our characters in there—the treating oncologist, the clinical investigator, the chaplain, the parents, the treating physician, the thoughtful and not-so-thoughtful scientists, the caretakers, and most importantly, the child. I had never read the description of a dying child or what goes on quite like this. This is Camus in the most non-existentialist mode one can be. You could say he believed in God. His first line is, "The only important question in life is whether or not you should commit suicide." In essence he drives the nail home, that if you've made the choice and decide not to commit suicide, then understand why you have made that choice.

It was very interesting and I don't quite know whether it did what I was hoping for it to do. I gave a lectureship called "The Robbie Hunton Lecture," which is on palliative care and how senior physicians can deal with that. It teaches them how to do medicine. I used *The Plague* to talk on what we are doing right and wrong about palliative care. It was a much more difficult talk for me to give. I am much more used to talking about chromative structure and targeted antibodies. I read from that section of *The Plague* and it still remains in my mind as one of the most appropriate pieces of literature. I think it is something that parents should look at. It is not easy stuff. Reading Camus is not easy, but it brings you to a different level of understanding as opposed to some of the other stuff that is out there. So, Albert Camus and I go back a long ways.

I do try to bring in important literature from people that are just a hell of a lot smarter than I am. *The Divine Comedy* is something that I read every year. Shakespeare, Lear, there are very few pieces of literature that deal with this subject in such non-judgmental and yet insightful ways. The Book of "Solomon" is extraordinary. "Genesis." Harold Bloom's book on wisdom writers (*Where Shall Wisdom Be Found?*; Riverhead Books) is a really excellent text to look at for good advice on good things to read. I think it comes out of your heritage, your background, what moves you. I always recommend people to go back to "the sacred texts"—and that does not mean religious texts exclusively.

I think that for families and for patients it is absolutely vital to have an involved mental health team. If you were to accept a patient with leukemia and did not have chemotherapy, I believe that would be a malpractice. I have viewed mental health services in the same way. If you have accepted a patient with cancer to treat, then it is your responsibility to have mental health services and help them. The people who do that work to help families make our job easier. The key is to have a team you can trust, where you can share things within a very personal way. There is nothing impersonal about these experiences.

I have an entire set of things, what we have called a "Day One Talk." It is when you sit down with the parents. It's never a talk, but a beginning of a relationship. One must be sure you are telling them that you have a definite diagnosis. I'll never forget, one time I was in Boston and one of my younger fellows went into a room. I said, "You can start this and I'll watch." There was a really, really husky father of this young girl we had diagnosed with leukemia. The fellow said, "We think your daughter has leukemia." The father grabbed him by the shirt around the neck and picked him up. The father said, "You think?" When you know, you know.

I try to tell people, "This will change your lives forever. It will not always necessarily change them in the worst way. It will change your lives in the short-term, interim and the long term." Once you have that in mind, I think it puts it in perspective.

I always try to make parents understand that it is nobody's fault. This is important to siblings as well. If they had a fight the previous day, they think it is related to the diagnosis.

It is really important to establish the playing field in terms of short-term and long-term objectives. People have to understand that as much as we know about the disease there are treatments that we may not know about. Percentages can help some people and can devastate others. They can also give false hope. You have to play the percentage game very carefully. You cannot cure somebody 50 percent. We always try to make people understand that while it is extremely important for them to know whether our treatment works or does not work, we are still going to take care of that child and them.

I try to tell medical students and residents and fellows that your job isn't just to cure people, it's to take care of them.

I explain that there are alternatives to therapy and different approaches on how the therapy arose. It is extremely important for individuals to enter themselves into a clinical trial. How to explain these trials is not an easy task.

Some parents will often say, I know this is not going to help my child, but I think it will help others. That's not a criteria to enroll a child into a study. The fact that a child cannot really be informed creates a situation where a parent has to give what we call vicarious consent, with the intent of benefiting that child.

I always tell people that if I would not put my own child on a treatment or clinical trial, I sure as hell would not be recommending it for them. We talk about side effects and goals of the therapy. Those goals vary depending upon the diagnosis.

There are some discussions that begin with, "Your child has almost a 100% chance of dying within twelve months. Let's figure out what we are going to do." So depending upon the diagnosis, the whole discussion can change profoundly.

I also tell people that they are going to have amazingly smart people thinking and worrying about their child. They all want the best for you and your child. They may not always say things in the same way and it may get confusing. Uncle Eddie in Des Moines may say, "Yeah, I knew somebody who got that and they did this." Or you may have somebody who lives three doors down who got something that your child is not getting. All of these questions are going to play a part. As soon as you are asking these questions to yourself, you have to sit down with your doctor and care team—nurse, physician assistant, so forth—and say, "I'm confused." I always try to keep that door completely open.

Just like the obligation to provide treatment and mental health services, the obligation to have a survivorship approach is also there. The side effects in the future will be different than the side effects we see now. The real challenge is for the people developing the therapies. We don't want bad late effects, but the worst and most common adverse late effect is a relapse of your cancer. Our biggest challenge is trying to fix the problem in the first place or, even better, preventing it.

Access to care is a hugely important issue, for care and for follow-up. I suspect that it is an untapped area of investigation. I don't think that we know the disparities of care in survivorship yet.

Science is a process of self-discovery and self-correction. I think that people have to understand this from their inner core up to their brain. It is very uncommon that what we would consider a major breakthrough translates into a curative breakthrough in a very short time. This (medical research) is an incredibly intense, time-consuming, humiliating and possibly the most extraordinary thing that anybody can experience.

The landscape has changed profoundly since when we started this movie. For instance, in pediatrics all of the four separate cooperative groups in North America have merged into one. I'm talking about clinical trial groups—they have united as The Children's Oncology Group. We can learn more from the databases and the sample collections when we have centralized registries. We can be more resourceful in our use of funds by having a singular group with a singular administration. We can improve the speed by which clinical trials are conceived, developed, executed and written up.

There is less money for research work than there was. This is an extraordinary tragedy. Because without commenting on the political realities in our lives these days, there's only so much money to go around. A heck of a lot of it is being put into things besides biomedical research.

It is national public health funding. The National Institutes of Health are and should be the engine that drives entrepreneurial and academic research. We have entered, and are growing deeper, in a time where government support for that kind of work has been severely cut back.

One criticism has been, "My God, you guys have gotten all this money in the past years and you still haven't cured cancer. Why do you deserve to continue to get the support?" This is more complicated than going to the moon. It's more complicated than going to Mars. Cancer is a heterogeneous disease. It is extremely resistant, and has extraordinary genetic instability that allows it to circumvent our best attempts to get rid of it. It is hard to detect early.

There are enormous values to early detection. That is not so easy in children, if a baby is born with leukemia. However, there are other tumors in adults and children that can probably be prevented. I hope that some day we can vaccinate children against leukemia so they won't get it. These are hopes that take people, time and money. This work is not cheap. I can assure you that these grants are not being used to buy Porsches. People are struggling to hire sufficient staff to do the experiments, to do the work, and to pay for the work. Then they need to develop those things into clinical discoveries that can be tested. That takes money. It takes generations of people. What I see happening, and I know I'm not the only one just saying this, is that we have a catastrophe in the making.

People could say that philanthropy, private biotechnology, and pharmaceutical support can make up the gap. They probably can't. They can help tremendously, but we need all three venues in order to make this work. There are some areas in pediatrics where you cannot engage a pharmaceutical company because the market is not going to be a payoff for them.

There have been a couple of companies that we have worked with and gotten drugs approved this last year for childhood leukemia, but it's rare that a company will focus on getting drug approval in a pediatric cancer. There are some areas where early drug development must be a partnership with academics, NIH and the FDA. That still takes money. No matter if you are doing it in eight hundred children or eight hundred thousand adults, those early trials still cost about the same.

I know people are trying to do the best thing, but there has never been a time when there is more important discovery work potentially available. There has never been a time where we are actually seeing the possibility of developing truly tumor-targeted therapies and putting them into practice. It's such an extraordinary opportunity. I know Albert Camus would be on our side. It's about the right fight. A society ultimately has to be judged on what it can do for it's sick, elderly and feeble. I suspect we have money, but we just have to use it the right way.

My time in this business, my own small way, I remain absolutely excited and I don't even want to sleep because of the potential of what we can do.

Chapter 7

Care GIVERS

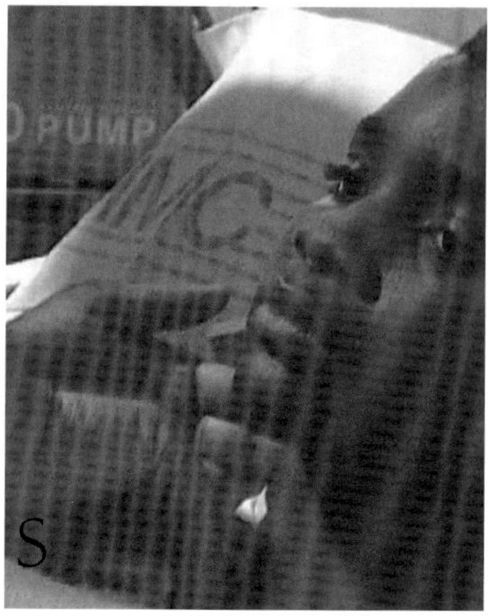

frederickHUANG, M.D.

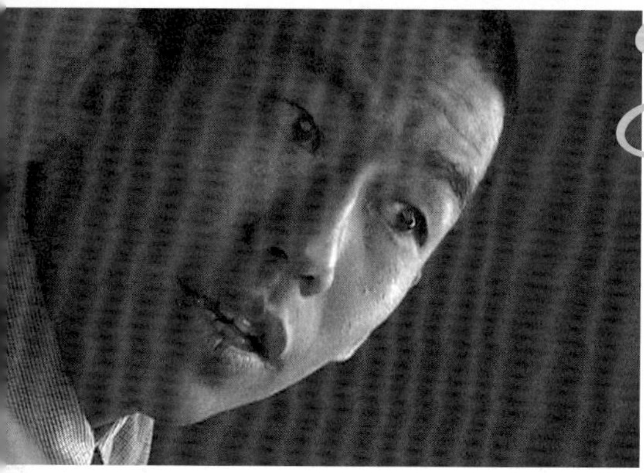

Dr. Fred Huang looking at Al's scans.

In addition to Dr. Arceci, there were several other medical professionals who cared for the children in A Lion in the House *at Cincinnati Children's Hospital Medical Center while the movie was being made. They shared their thoughts on a number of key issues raised in the film. These professionals and their current positions are:*

Vinod V. Balasa, M.D. Assistant Professor of Pediatrics and Director of the Thrombophilia Program in the Hemophilia and Thrombosis Center of the hematology/oncology division at Cincinnati Children's Hospital Medical Center.

Cynthia DeLaat, M.D. Medical director of the ATP Five-Plus Clinic for cancer survivors at Cincinnati Children's Hospital Medical Center. Inspired by her travel to Guatemala where she did volunteer community medical service, Dr. Delaat devotes much of her time to working with predominantly Hispanic immigrants at an urban Babies' Milk Fund Clinic.

Frederick Huang, M.D. Director of the Department of Pediatric Hematology and Oncology at The University of Texas Medical branch in Galveston.

Paul Jubinsky, M.D., Ph.D. Assistant Professor of Pediatric Hematology and Oncology, at the Albert Einstein College of Medicine at Yeshiva University, New York.

Connie Koons R.N., B.S.N. Charge nurse in the blood and marrow transplant unit of the hematology/oncology division at Cincinnati Children's Hospital Medical Center.

Linda Polman, R.N., B.S.N. Education coordinator for inpatient and outpatient nursing staff in the hematology/oncology division at Cincinnati Children's Hospital Medical Center.

Theodore Zwerdling, M.D. Associate Professor, Pediatric Hematology/Oncology, University of California Davis Medical Center, Sacramento CA.

On making A Lion in the House:

BALASA: Frankly, the presence of the cameras did not affect my behavior or my interactions with the patients or the families, and I have never regretted taking part in the project.

DELAAT: At the very beginning, I felt uncomfortable. I don't like to be on camera, period. You'd start to begin a pretty serious conversation, and the camera would come around. I remember one time at the beginning I was doing a spinal tap on a patient. She was upset and all of a sudden a microphone comes flying over my head. It was a little bit startling. But after a few weeks, Julia and Steve were so professional, the families were obviously comfortable, and you didn't even notice that the cameras were there. They are really good at what they do.

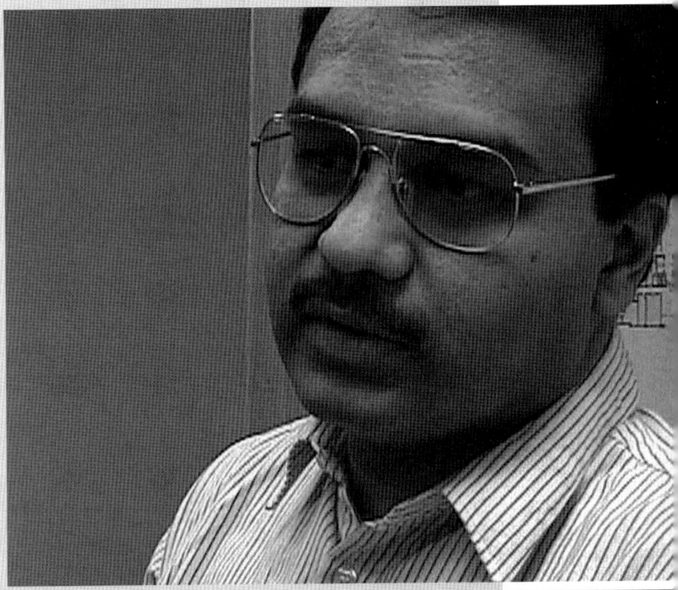

Dr. Vinod Balasa concerned.

HUANG: My relationship with Julia and Steve started very shortly after I got to Cincinnati in 1997 as a pediatric hematology/oncology fellow at Children's. I happened to be involved in the care of a child, Al Fields, who they had chosen to feature in this film. Like a lot of people I was acutely aware of the camera at first. What they say is true; you just forget it is there.

In a scene early in the movie I was addressing a resident about a particular patient; I still look at that scene and feel a little badly about it. I don't think I was inappropriate, but I was certainly very stern. I think that I had reason to be stern. I think that is a good example of how I was honestly not inhibited by the cameras. If I had been, I would have taken the time to speak in a different tone, but I didn't.

JUBINSKY: To me, the movie meant creating a realistic depiction of what families go through, one that would be beneficial to the families and the people who interact with them. The cameras were slightly distracting. How one interacts in "public" is different than how you do in private. There is awareness that what you say or do might be interpreted differently by an outside observer than by someone who knows you well, such as the family and staff. It was definitely a worthwhile endeavor.

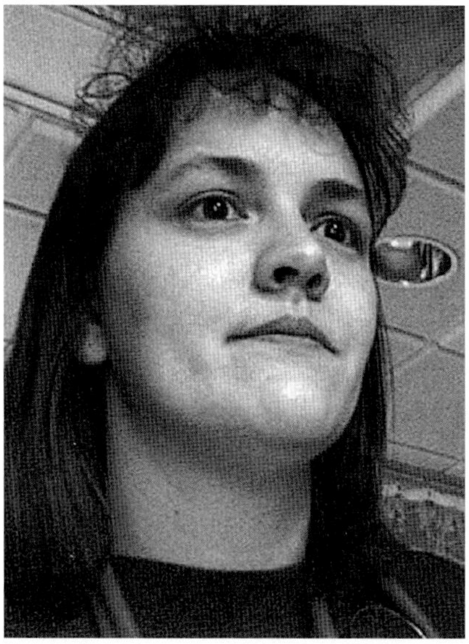
Tim's nurse, Connie Koons.

KOONS: We were given a rationale for the presence of the cameras and it seemed like a good cause, so I did not mind the cameras being around on the unit. I felt if it would get out to others that cancer affects families and the patient in different ways and that it is not necessarily a death sentence, then it was worth having the cameras around.

Having the cameras on the unit and taping all of the time did feel intrusive at times. There were times that staff just wanted to sit down and eat lunch and be able to talk, and the next thing you know there was a camera in your face. I did not particularly care to be taped while I was eating.

As far as affecting my behavior with my interactions with the patients and families, it did not.

I pride myself in the care I give and do not change that care, no matter who is watching. I have no regrets in taking part in the taping. I am very much looking forward to seeing the final product. The kids in the video touched all of the nurses lives in different ways and I was pretty close to a couple of the kids and their families.

POLMAN: Eventually I blocked the cameras out of my mind and concentrated on what I was doing. I thought more of remaining as honest as possible and optimistic about the patient's outcome My interaction with families was the same whether the camera was present or not on any given day. I have no regrets at all in taking part in the project. I am proud that I am a part of something so intimate and was able to relate to these families. They became part of my family too, and it seems like only yesterday that the experience happened. I'm not sure I want to relive those days and I'm sure it will be hard for the families to see this film.

On what parents need to know when their children are diagnosed with cancer:

BALASA: The most important thing is to remember that while cancer treatment is difficult, most children do very well and are cured of their cancer.

DELAAT: The older kids going through this have the same emotions as the parents. I think some family members try to protect the older children with cancer. I don't know that that is the best thing to do. The adolescent needs to express his or her fears, worries, and sad times like everybody else. Families think the kid is sick and they do not want to burden them more. I think a child worries more. You need to give them an opportunity to know and say how they feel.

The other thing I would say is take things one day at a time. Take it in small pieces. Take it one step at a time and don't be overwhelmed.

HUANG: It is important for people to know that they are not alone. I mean that very broadly. It is not just the doctors and nurses that will be taking care of their child. There are psychologists, social workers, health educators, physical therapists, occupational therapists and a whole host of people who are very good at what they do. I think that families often have problems they try to handle on their own, not knowing that we could identify tons of folks on the team who would be capable of addressing them.

Once the news settles in, parents realize that there are other kids and other families there. There is often shared ground; that can be very, very helpful. There are organizations dedicated to making sure that these newly diagnosed children and their families are made aware of resources. This is not a journey that they have to take alone. There will be a lot of people on their side rooting for them.

JUBINSKY: They are not alone, they will make it through the ordeal, and that there will be many changes in their lives, both for better and worse. For all, I strongly suggest that this is a time when the family needs to pull together in the same direction.

KOONS: The best people to help the family get the support they need are our social work team. They have a vast knowledge of the resources available to the families. The staff at the hospital are there to help the parents as much as they are there to treat the child. Other parents who are going through the same thing can be a great resource for them as well.

POLMAN: This is a very long journey ahead of them, and it is like a roller coaster with many ups and downs. You will become extremely knowledgeable about your child's disease. Take each day at a time and enjoy the little pleasures in life with your child and family.

ZWERDLING: I can't think of one aspect of the parent's and child's life that is not going to change. There's certainly the mechanical things—taking care of a catheter, learning to do sterile technique at home, giving all the meds, knowing when to call the doctor. They end up with skills that nurses would envy. They have to deal with the fact that their child has changed in body habit. The children lost their hair; they've lost weight, The family has to know how to react. Who do they tell and when do they tell? Do they tell the neighbor? Do they tell the teacher? It's every single thing from when you get up until you go to sleep at night and most likely in your dreams as well.

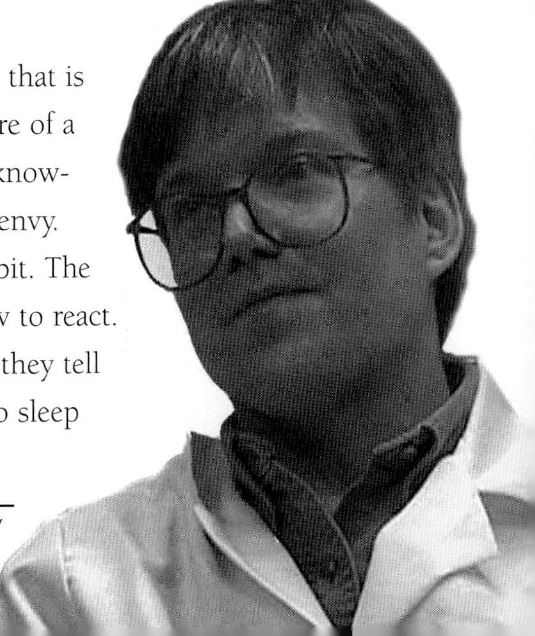

Dr. Paul Jubinsky

On relationships with patients and families:

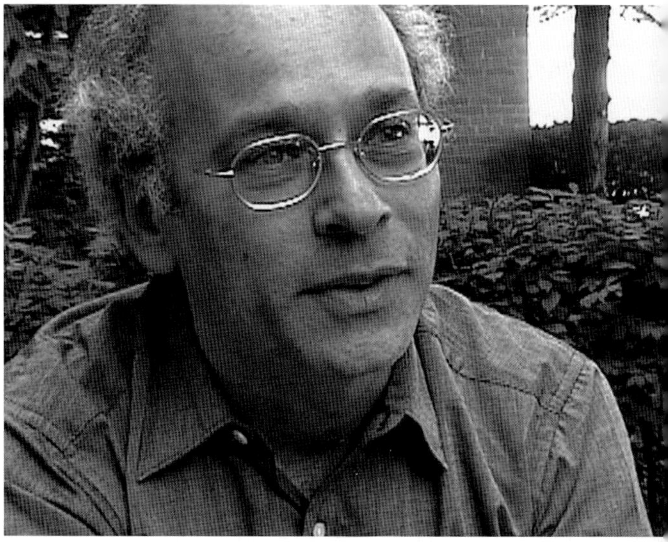

Dr. Ted Zwerdling

HUANG: The culture of medicine nowadays mandates that we inform our patients. We have become much more open in letting families know what they are buying into for their child.

When I sit down with families, I still struggle to this very day to figure out the best balance between not giving them enough information versus saying, "If you are going to agree to all this medicine, then you need to agree to every little side effect, rare or common, severe or minor."

What may happen is, it will overwhelm the parents. There are wonderful studies that show that parents getting news like that retain very little of what they are told. They may nod and smile and repeat back what they have heard, but they truly did not understand. Repetition is the key. So I go over that the first time and make sure they understand the really big side effects, and quickly go over the more rare side effects, and then repetition, repetition, repetition. The more they hear it, the more they will remember, understand it, and put it in context.

I am a big believer that the patient-physician relationship is very much about the personal relationship. My assignment to Al Fields in oncology was purely random. It just happened that I was up on the rotation, but we had a great relationship. We understood each other.

The oncologist is the team leader. I make it my point to be informed about what is going on, so when I go to the parents, I can tie it altogether for them about what is going on with their kid.

One of the joys for me as a pediatrician is that I do get to work with families. To me, that is very gratifying. It is how healthcare ought to be, that whole family approach.

KOONS: I love what I do. I love the kids and I love the interaction with the kids and the families, I love watching the families grow, and learn as they go. Going from a new diagnosis where the family is scared out of their mind saying I can't do this there's no way, to weeks later, to months later, to doing a really good job, and they're telling me about it, and explaining different things to me and understand every bit of it. And knowing that I have been a part of helping them grow and get to where they are now. A lot of what we do is very intense, but I love what I do.

ZWERDLING: This work allows you an intimacy that very few other areas of medicine allow. You can deal with people pretty much as they are. You don't have to worry about what they think you're going to be, what you're supposed to be, what you're supposed to look like. You can come in and sit down and discuss things with them, and you get to know them really well in an extreme situation. So a lot of the blinders, a lot of the facades that people have, are not operating because their child is affected with something that is life-threatening. And because you're going to be with them for a long period of time.

Dealing with cancer is a long-term commitment. When we take care of somebody we will take care of them for many years, or for the rest of their life. So we really get to know the children and the families and the patients. You have to be careful. There are times when you have to remember that you're the physician; you're not a buddy. This can be a big problem with physicians and nurses, to know where the boundaries are. You're there to make medical decisions, and to communicate with them in a manner that people understand, and in a compassionate manner. But you're not there to be people's friend—and that means making difficult decisions, unpopular decisions.

When you're in the hospital for a long time, you can have a group of people who are going in one direction and twenty-four hours later the direction can be completely different. Especially at the resident level, it's very difficult for parents at a teaching hospital to have to put up with all the personalities, all the changes. Pediatric oncology carries a lot of baggage with it and not everybody is suited to deal with the intensity of the situation. A lot of times that comes across as being abrupt or being cold. Most of the time it's not. It's just lack of experience and anxiety on the part of the physician who is caring for a very sick child.

When you come out of medical school, you really have a maternal model of looking at things. You are providing information, you are providing care, you're treating people, you touch them, you ask them intimate questions. As time goes on, I have become much more of a person to provide information and help people make difficult decisions, but not as a mother or a father or a friend would. More somebody who has a particular expertise that can allow decisions to be made, but not to be demanding or overpowering.

So I think there's been a huge change. Actually I feel much healthier about it. There's a lot less burden. It's not us making the decision—"This is what you will do." It's us helping you get to a point to make a good decision for your child. So there's not the burden of being always right, always all-encompassing. Some of it is part of the new consumerism. People want to be part of a decision-making processes. They want to take command and control of some things. To a degree, I think that is beneficial because it allows everybody to work as a team, as a unit. However, sometimes it swings too far and parents try and dictate. It happens, and it happens more and more as time goes on. It's hard for families to know exactly how and at what level to be making these decisions. It's not just reading a website, which some people think it is.

On confronting the end of a child's life:

DeLaat: What I have always told parents is just to trust their gut about what feels right. We try to present options, from very aggressive to doing nothing to everything in between that may be a benefit for their child. If they keep coming back to, "I want to do everything possible" then that is what we need to try to do, if it is something that has a chance of working and benefiting their child. You don't just keep pulling drugs off the shelf to do something. I have had children live six months in situations where I never predicted that. I think parents end up making the right decisions.

Another thing, I know when the child cannot be cured the parents have to be there to pick up the pieces of the rest of their lives when the child dies. They have to feel they did what was right for their child. They have to be at peace that they did what was best for their child, no matter what the outcome. I think kids know for the most part that they are going to be okay when they die. I think they are most concerned about what is going to happen to their parents and their siblings because they know they are not going to be there.

Some of the most challenging, heart-wrenching times for me is telling a teenager that they are not going to survive their illness. You don't have a conversation like that with a four or five year old. It is hard when you have to sit down with a sixteen year old and tell him that this is the third time your cancer has come back and we don't have anything that is going to cure you.

We never got trained in this. I sought out advice from chaplains and psychologists that I got to know over the years. You do learn from experience, but it is something that I think you can always do better.

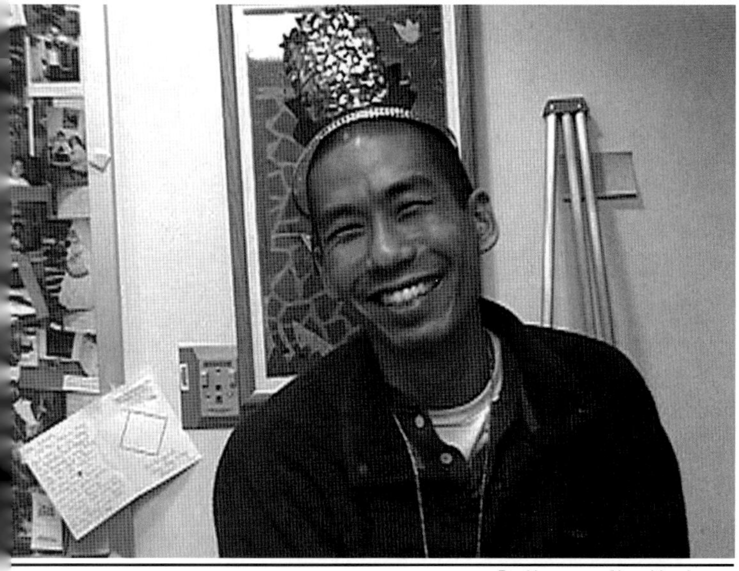

Dr. Huang on New Year's eve.

HUANG: How do you help parents decide when it is time to stop treament? It's really hard. Certainly the child is number one, and the decisions need to be focused on that child. However, it is not as simple as that. There are ramifications for any decision that you make for your child that you are going to have to live with for a much longer time. The child, no matter what the outcome, is going to be taken care of. What I try to say to my families is they have to think about what that decision is going to mean to them. They have to be okay with that decision five, ten and twenty years down the line.

JUBINSKY: Believe me, kids know what death is. They know what it is to die. I've had a lot of kids tell me, "Don't tell mom that I'm doing really bad, I don't want her to know that I'm sick. I think I'm dying. Don't tell mom because she's going to get really upset and she's going to cry." They are amazing in what they really do. When things are bad, you never hear any of them complaining. They want to be tough for everybody else.

POLMAN: My frustration is empowering the families too much, with too much information, too much decision-making. Those are all ethical issues, and a lot of our kids end up not having a dignified death. I personally strive for a dignified death, as much as you can have in the hospital, without too many heroics, and going too far, then having to make the decision to withdraw. That's not a good decision to have to make either. To stop treatment, and literally have to pull the plug; it's agonizing. If there is a chance for survival, then give them that chance. But if it's extremely slim, why put the family through it? When you get to that point, why give them still more hope?

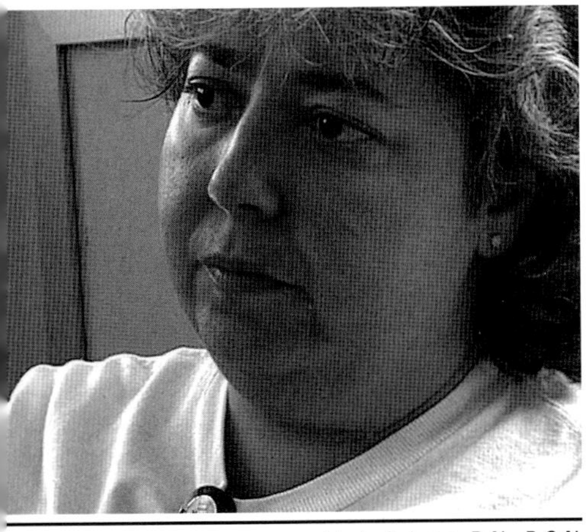

Linda Polman, R.N., B.S.N.

ZWERDLING: The physician has the obligation to let parents know what can be done. There is also the obligation to tell parents what you think should be done. And those two are usually very different. If it's hard for us, it's impossible for the families. You just have to keep supporting them, making sure they know what your opinion is, but always honoring their desires. I don't think there is a good way to die, but I think there are things that can make death bad. Frequently, when death is coming, it's not the enemy anymore. The cancer, the disease process is the enemy, and alleviating suffering is far more important than trying yet another futile attempt at treatment.

On the state of medicine:

BALASA: Things are developing at a breakneck speed in the field, with new advances and improvements occurring in all aspects of diagnosis and therapy. There are several new drugs that are better with fewer side effects and there have also been improvements in supportive care.

DELAAT: Because childhood cancer is a relatively rare disease, most insurance companies will cover experimental therapy. It may take a little bit of effort on the physician's part, if we can get to talk to another physician to say, "This is why I think this is appropriate for this child." We are not just saying, "Let's do a bone marrow transplant because there is nothing else to do." If we can prove it has been done with a reasonable chance of success, most of the time those are approved. One in ten thousand kids get cancer each year. How many thousands of adults have heart disease? It's not like everybody is knocking on their door for these therapies. I think that it is also because it is a child. If the child gets better, there are many more productive years left for that child. I think for the most part insurance companies have been very reasonable with us.

HUANG: There is no doubt overall that we have made some incredible advances. It's not just about medicine, but the other things that we do—for example, nausea control or pain control, the emotional, psychological and spiritual health as well.

Childhood cancer isn't the death trap that people think it is. We do much better with children than an oncologist with an adult cancer patient. I would never wish cancer on anyone, but it is not a "throw in the towel, there is nothing we can do" scenario. I am encouraged by the progress we have made because I only see that we are going to get much, much better with it.

People in my position fifty years from now may think that everything I did was the old dark, stone-age days. "They gave chemotherapy, they actually injected poisonous drugs into their veins. What were they thinking?"

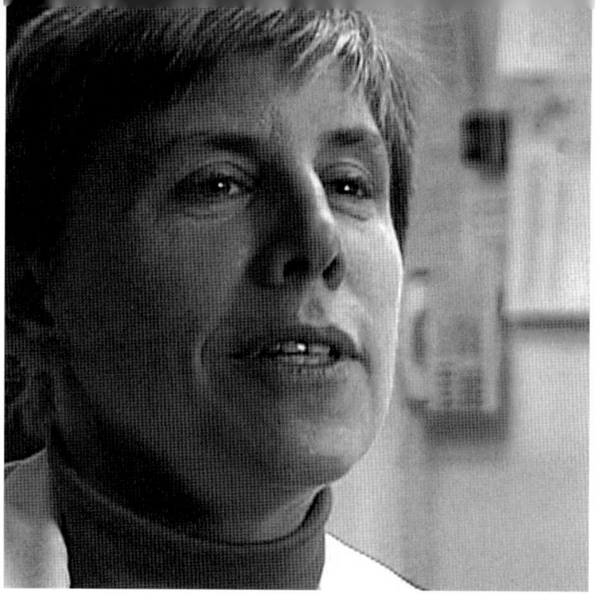

Dr. Cyndi DeLaat

I really hope one day technology and advances and discovery and research and learning get to a point where we can say that about what I did. Wouldn't that be wonderful? You could go into an office and get a drug with no toxicity that would cure you of your disease, whether that be cancer, arthritis, diabetes.

I'm not only hopeful, I am almost certain that there will come a day where cancer will be something we can take care of effectively, permanently, and with minimum side effects. I'm confident that that day will come.

On survivorship:

Because of her work at the survivors' clinic at Cincinnati Children's, Dr. Delaat is particularly well versed in the issues that follow cancer survivors into adolescence and adulthood.

Our estimates are that one in nine hundred kids who are twenty to twenty-five years of age is a cancer survivor. That is a lot.

We see kids who were probably treated in the '70s and early '80s who have problems with fertility, meaning that they are not able to have kids. We have kids who have problems with other endocrine issues; women can have premature menopause, men can have inadequate testosterone production.

The survivors are very resilient psychologically. There are some kids who have post-traumatic stress symptoms or are preoccupied with their health. I would say that is the minority. We have a lot of kids choosing to do things in the medical field, nursing, physical therapy. There are a lot of kids in our clinic particularly in medical school. I don't know if their cancer experience has influenced them to want to help people, somewhat like other people who helped them get through their illness.

Some of these kids do struggle, particularly those who had therapy directed towards the central nervous system. They have problems with learning. We recognize that and have a school intervention program to assist the families to get the kids help in school that they need.

Fifteen years ago when we started our clinic, it was more difficult to get the kids the help that they need. Now actually some colleges even have specific programs for learning-disabled kids and recognize that cancer survivors potentially would need their services. It can take a lot of effort. That is why we have a person who is well versed to tell these families how to get the help they need.

Over the last ten years in most pediatric centers that treat children with cancer, long-term follow-up clinics have sprung up. We have had ours since 1988. The problem is how do you get this knowledge to the people who see these kids every day or to the young adults who never come back to a survivor clinic?

There are two hurdles: 1) We are just gathering that knowledge so that we have an understanding that if a child had this type of cancer with these treatments these are the risks. We are systematically evaluating these survivors. 2) How do you get this knowledge to the survivor and the primary care community? That is kind of where things are at right now.

When I work at our survivor clinic, I see primary care physicians all the time. Anytime there is a problem with the child, the primary physician blames it on the chemo the child received. That is not true. They get the same illnesses that everybody else gets. If we had a better way of getting this knowledge to the medical community, then they would feel more comfortable with these kids. I think The Childrens' Oncology Group is starting to focus a little bit more on this. They have guidelines on their website on how these kids should be evaluated.

It is a focus I think that needs to continue to grow to get this knowledge out to the people who take care of these kids on a day-to-day basis.

Making THE FILM

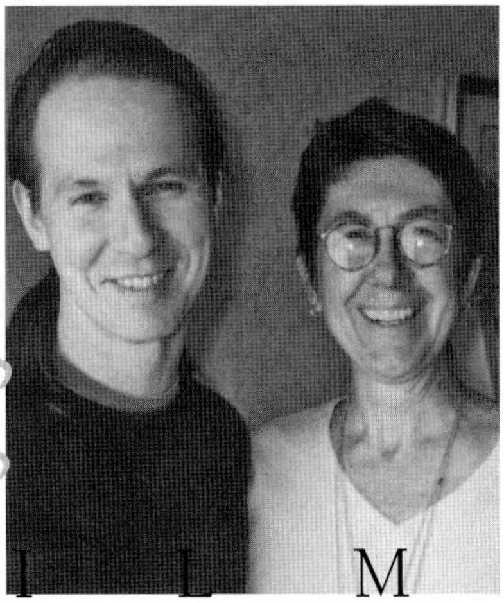

Steven Bognar & Julia Reichert, in the early days of shooting the film.

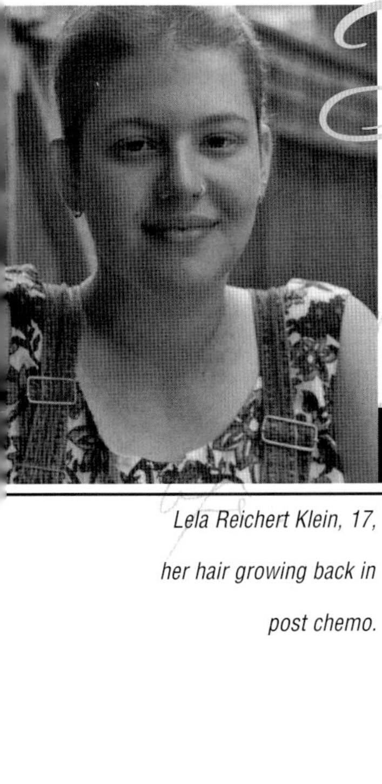

Lela Reichert Klein, 17, her hair growing back in post chemo.

Filmmakers' Journal

This chapter weaves together stories and memories from LION directors Steven Bognar & Julia Reichert, editors Mary Lampson, Jaime Meyers, Ann Rotolante and production team members Melissa Godoy, Karen Durgans & Dan Misch.

gettingSTARTED

JULIA REICHERT:

My daughter Lela was diagnosed with a relatively rare cancer, lymphoma, in 1996, a week before her seventeenth birthday. This plunged us both into the most harrowing and painful year and a half of our lives. I know the shock and disorientation parents feel. I've faced the huge decisions that must be made on a dime. I've sat up night after night, reading everything available on cancer, day after day, watching my lively girl turn sick and gray.

I've felt the helplessness that must quickly turn to a will of iron. I know what it is like to have one clear focus in life: the survival of my child. I also know from observation the suffering of the children, not only the great physical pain involved in cancer treatment, but the psychic pain of losing hair, losing friends, giving up on school and most normal childhood activities.

And yet, with time's perspective, I see the positive side. My daughter is fine. In my almost sixty years I have never faced anything as challenging or, ironically, as rewarding. I see the tremendous bonds that can develop between parent and child, brother and sister, caregiver and patient.

Through my experience with her, deepened by making this film, I see the untapped wells of love, patience and strength that are waiting within us. And above all, I am continually amazed by the resilience of the children. If this film can capture just a fraction of all this, it can begin to live up to its potential.

I would never have considered taking on this film if I had not, myself, gone through the experience of fighting cancer with my child. Otherwise, I would see myself as a voyeur, peering into other people's heartache. Instead, my life gave me a goal: To help to end the isolation of people fighting cancer.

When Steve and I walked into those hospital rooms and the parents heard our story, the walls fell down right away. The other parents were full of empathy, curiosity (What did she have? What treatment did she get? How is she now?) and encouragement.

I am a member of the same community as the moms in our film. As such, I saw my role as a participant as well as observer, and, perhaps even more, as a witness to profound events.

For my entire adult life, I have seen myself as a social issue filmmaker. I am very proud of my past work. Yet I hope *Lion* may be seen as the most political of all, because it so deeply reveals what we in the human family are made of.

Julia's Journal, Sunday, January 14, 11:20 AM

"It's still snowing. Piles of white everywhere. But everything is totally different. It's sunny today. The snow is melting for the second day. The nightmarish moments of blizzard in recent days are gone in the sparkly sunlight.

But my chest is tight and I am very scared. How to even write this down? Lela may have cancer. It looks like it. We found out a few days after my last entry. Lymphoma. I feel very guilty. And scared. And scared for her. We don't know for sure yet. But if it's not lymphoma, it's something else scary. She doesn't know. It is so hard, so odd, to hear her talk, knowing what I know. She's worried. She's worried she may have mono, etc. Yesterday she told me a story. She was talking with her friend Anna, who she hadn't seen in several months. Lela was going on and on about how angry she is. Why am I so angry? Who am I angry with? Anna finally said she was angry with her body. Lela said "Yeah, that's it. My body has been keeping me from doing things. From doing what I want, what I can." She knows she is sick. She's probably known it a lot longer than we have. It may be a year already. For sure the past few months. This helps explain her grades."

STEVEN BOGNAR:

We started shooting with just one digital video camera, a Sony VX-1000. At that time we didn't have a microphone, no wide angle lens, no boom pole or even headphones. But you can't let stuff stop you from making your movie. If you let the fact of not having a certain piece of equipment stop you from getting started, you're making excuses. We started shooting, and calling friends to see if we could borrow this or that. And little by little we began fumbling our way forward into having a professional set up. At first we had a microphone cable between the camera and the sound person. We were tethered. But it was absurd—we kept getting tangled up with each other, and worse, getting doctors entangled too. Those meeting rooms were crowded, and it's not cool to suddenly be making the residents trip over your mic cable. Our friend and colleague, Dan Friedman, loaned us his radio mic, which helped a lot. So much so that we ended up keeping it for the next four years!

Eventually we had this set up: A camera that had a cardioid microphone on top. A

Julia's Journal, on the plane, returning early from Sundance in 1966 to fight daughter Lela's cancer. Flying above the earth. Flying above anything solid. The solid below is frozen. It's ice. There are odd ravines, wrinkled scars. Inexplicable patterns. Nature knows. I cannot. Am I flying above my daughter's brain, that has told her cells to run amok. Or are those the surfaces of the malignancy, the runaway cells, the cancer? I want to ride over them on a fast horse, in battle gear, ready to strike any damned cell that dares to attack. I will defend my daughter.

Now the earth is like the fine veins in the neck, the chest over milky skin. Like Lela's milky chest, her white fine neck, skin luminescent, tender, so live. A proud neck, a beautiful head. Her upper chest & shoulders are spectacular. All this is where the cancer has been hiding. And now it is silently moving inside her proud neck"

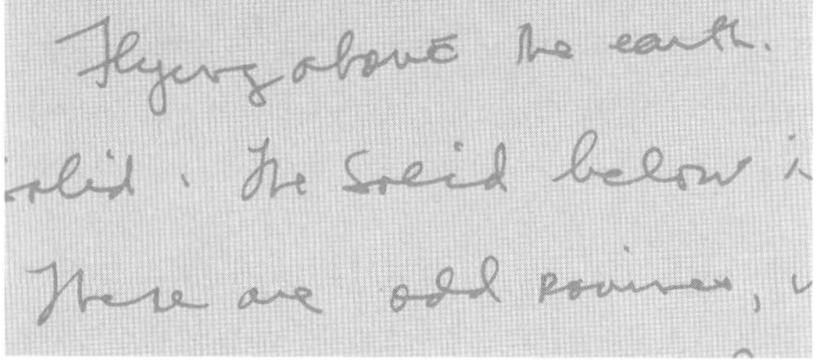

cardioid mic records sound in a heart shaped pattern, where the tip of the mic is the pointy bottom of the heart. The field of sound bulbs out from that kind of mic. It's good for hearing people within, say, five feet of the camera.

We then had a shotgun mic, on a boom pole. A boom pole is like a collapsible fishing pole, with a mic on the end—these are the things you see on TV news, with the furry blimp on the end, chasing down crooked politicians. We didn't use the furry blimp thingee, which cuts down wind noise, because we were indoors, and we wanted to keep our equipment as small and undistracting as possible.

Now, some sound recordists will argue that a boom pole should not have a shotgun mic on it. A shotgun microphone records sounds like a telescope sees—narrowly but with the ability to record far-away sounds. If you are aiming a shotgun mic properly, it can record decent sound from across a room. So why would you put it on a boom pole, which can get quite close to people? Why not use another cardioid mic on the boom pole?

In a lot of the doctor rounds meetings, or family meetings, having the shotgun on a boom pole was important, because many people are speaking from different places in a room, and there's no time to tip-toe over to them. If you have to walk over to whoever is speaking, you'll miss way too much. Conversation flies in real life, and people overlap. A boom pole hovers in the air, above the conversation, able to slide around. The key we learned was how to pivot the shotgun mic quickly so it was aimed in the right direction. After it was aimed, the boom could slowly be eased closer to that person. As long as we learned to immediately and silently pivot the mic, our sound was generally good.

The final component to our equipment was a radio mic. A radio mic is a small box that people clip to their belt, or put in their pocket. A wire comes out of the box and goes up to a tiny clip mic that people wear on their collar. We would ask parents, docs and sometimes kids to wear the mic—whoever we guessed would be talking the most that day. With one key person wearing the radio mic,

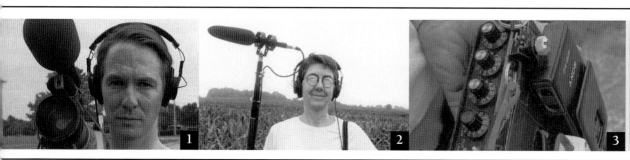

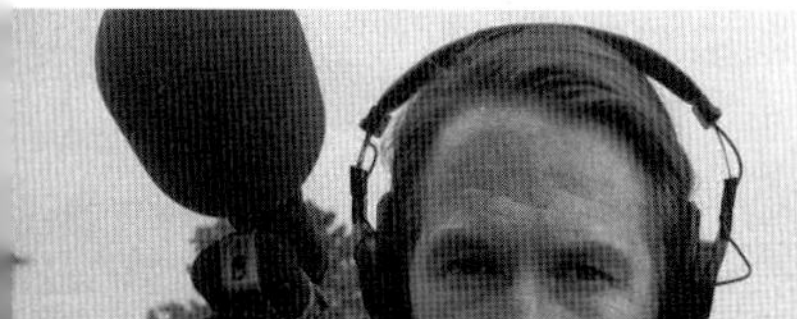
1

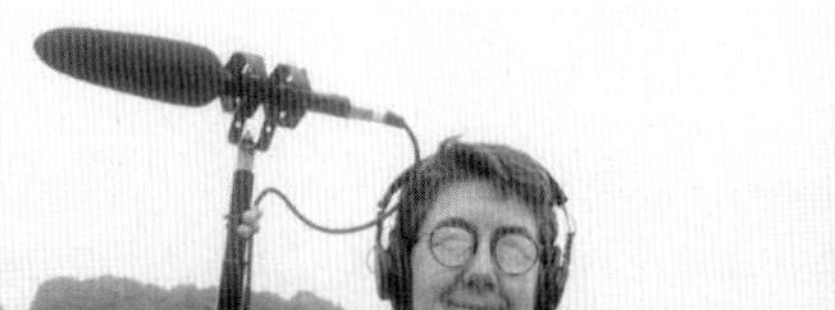
2

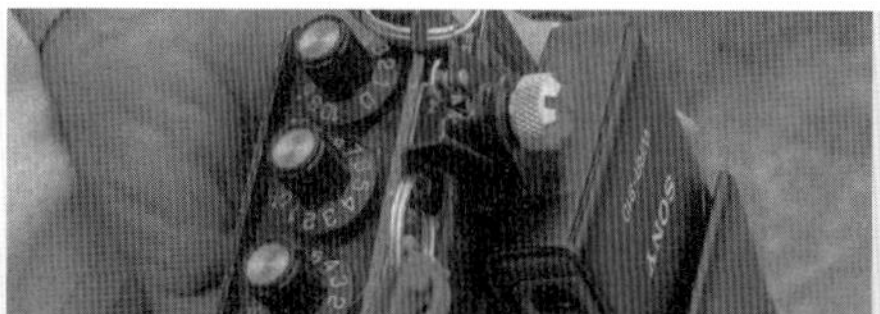
3

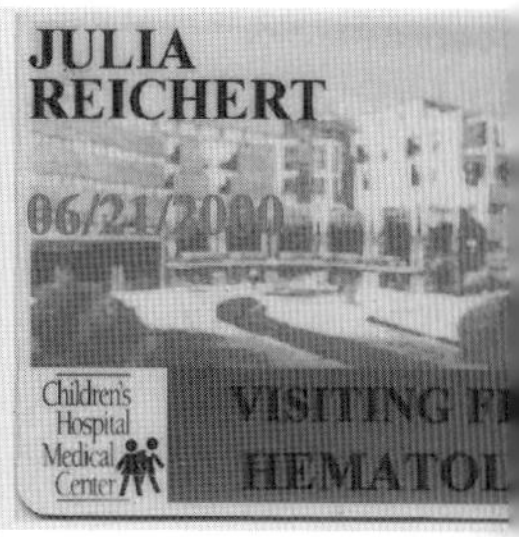
JULIA
REICHERT
06/21/2000
Children's Hospital Medical Center
VISITING F
HEMATOL

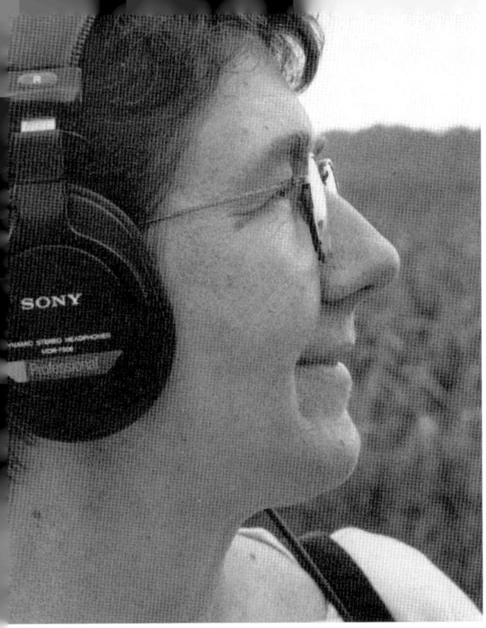

Julia Reichert wearing headphones. At first, the camera, boom pole and head phones seem odd to people in the film, but pretty quickly, people begin looking past the technology to see the filmmakers as individuals.

we didn't have to worry about swinging the boom pole over to them all the time. I wish we had had 3 radio mics, really. Good sound is so crucial to any film, and to documentary especially. Having good sound is far more important than having a good picture, because the story is more told by the sound. An audience will forgive a shaky bit of camera work. But they won't forgive a film if the sound is unintelligible.

JULIA:

We started making the drive to Cincinnati on a regular basis. At first the hospital had a staff person with us when we were filming. Usually it was Beth Cullen Canarie, who works for the Heme-Onc division as their school intervention staff person. She goes to the schools of their patients and explains a great deal to the classmates and teachers of a kid with cancer. She demystifies cancer, dispels myths, and it really helps a kid feel less out of place in their school. Beth would hang out with us during the filming, but after a few months, the hospital felt comfortable with us, almost everyone got to know us, and we were given Children's Hospital ID badges, for those who didn't know us.

One of the trying things about making this film was how isolated it made us from our friends and families. It was impossible to talk about it, because almost no one could understand what we were observing, what we were living through. We couldn't really explain it until we started having stuff we could show. Our friends didn't really know what we were going through until we had a rough cut screening, five years after we had started. Then they knew.

Most people, when they ask you what you're working on and we say, "We're making a film about kids fighting cancer," they say, "Oh, that must be really hard. I could never do that." It was a real conversation stopper. Of course, none of them had met the kids, met the families.

The film was something that Steve and I intensely shared. And I know it drew us much closer together. We were like the two hobbits who went the distance, and no one could know what it was. I remember when we started doing screenings. It was such a relief, that our friends could finally know what we'd been through. Same with the folks at ITVS, I had that same reaction.

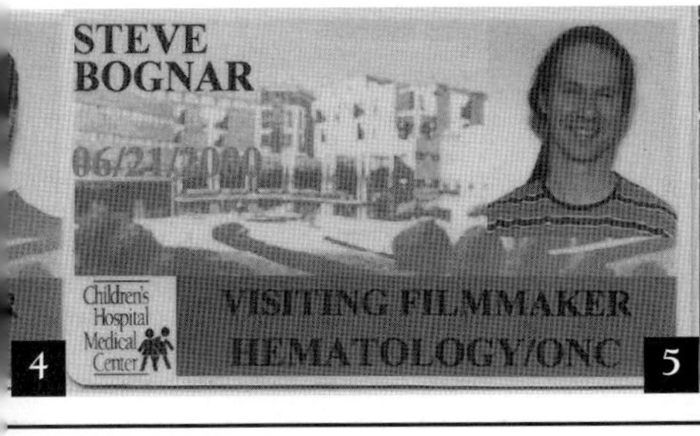

4 5

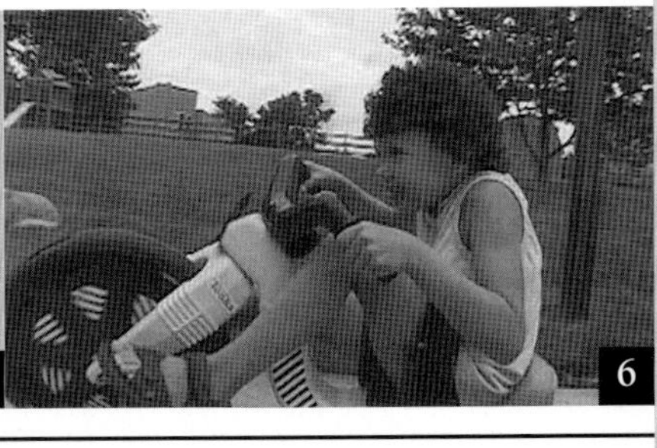

6

1 & 2. Steve & Julia would always wear headphones; both had to know the sound was good.

3. The audio gear: A Shure mixer (with the five knobs), a radio receiver to record the sound of whoever was wearing the radio microphone, and a small white transmitter box, which sent the sound to the camera.

4 & 5. Julia and Steve's ID badges from Cincinnati Children's. They were particularly fond of the "Visiting Filmmaker" title.

6. The first day of filming A Lion in the House. *Alex Lougheed racing around on her bigwheels with her little sister Jackie.*

STEVEN:

In the early days of filming, we argued a lot, about how to do this work. It was actually kind of bumpy.

JULIA:

We had different ideas of how we should be as filmmakers in the room—how we should be, what we should shoot. I remember the central question as how much should we be a "fly on the wall," staying out of the way, vs. how much do we interact. I thought we shouldn't be interacting a lot, and Steve thought we should—that we would be like normal people, except we would have cameras and be shooting.

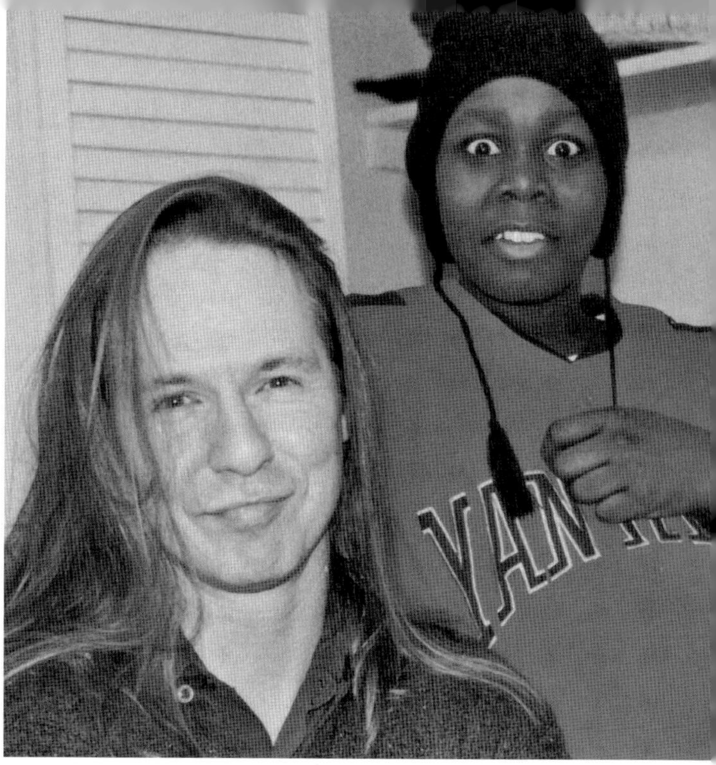

Al Fields reacts to the unruly length of Steve's hair. The next year, it would all fall out as Steve developed Alopecia, an auto-immune condition that causes a person to lose their hair. Some of the kids in the film said, "now you look like us."

STEVEN:

We also disagreed about how long to stay at someone's house, or in their hospital room. I was always hyper-self-conscious about overstaying our welcome. And I felt like Julia always wanted to stay way longer than people wanted us there. And you know, in Ohio, where people are generous and polite, they wouldn't tell us to leave. But I remember having a few big arguments in the car on the way home about how we should have left earlier, or how we should have stayed longer.

JULIA:

Steve was right in terms of the interactivity, and I was right in the need to stay. The thing I learned a lot from Steve was the need to be there, to interact, to bring coffee, food, little things.

STEVEN:

And I learned from Julia that we shouldn't leave when people got tired or cranky or whatever—that was part of what we were supposed to be documenting. It was part of a larger process for me in learning how not to flinch, as a documentarian—as a witness.

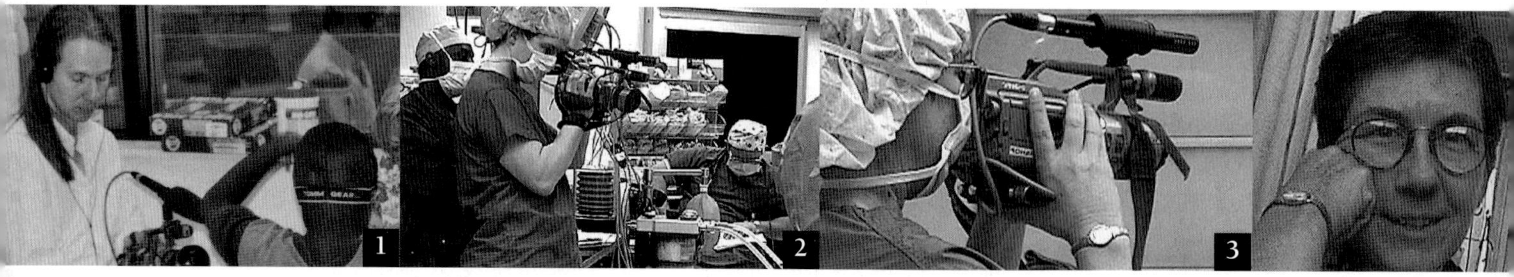

JULIA:

Early on, one of the first scenes we filmed, was of Jen Moone getting a spinal tap. It was very challenging, yet inspiring. That she could count to three, that she could go through that procedure, that she got up, wiped her face, that within a few minutes she was playing. It inspired me that Jen took control over scary stuff by playing with it. By playing with her medical supplies, her doctor kit, she made the spinal tap less scary.

STEVEN:

That moment was a turning point for me, in life and in this film. All my life, I've passed out whenever I'm watching an injection, getting a shot, even seeing needles being used in movies. I pass out cold. Like *Drugstore Cowboy*, Julia was with me—I would just know it's going to happen, so I slump down in my seat, and black out. A few moments later, I come to. But that's how strong my needle phobia has been. So here we are shooting Jen's spinal tap, which in the movie is less than a minute long, but which in real life went on for over 20 minutes. And it got harder and harder, seeing that needle hovering, hearing her screaming. Julia was crying, as she held the boom pole. And I started getting very lightheaded. But it was one of those moments in life, when you have to ask yourself, are you up for the task. And so I didn't pass out, and now I don't have a needle phobia anymore.

JULIA:

Making a film in hand-held cinema verité was a tough, wonderful, personal challenge. Neither of us had worked in this way, as a two-person crew, with the ability to keep shooting—I mean literally rolling tape—hour after hour. Sheer endurance was a factor for me at times. I was over 50 when we started. The physical demands of holding the camera or boom pole were great. Would I be able to come through? Looking back, I'm proud that I was able to do it. I don't think I ever seriously considered giving up on the project. We didn't want to be anywhere else in the world. It was always the most compelling thing in our lives, a rare privilege. Yet it was something we couldn't really describe to our friends and family. It really became an experience we shared only with the families, the nurses and docs, and each other. That's one reason why this film really drew us together.

Our learning curve wasn't just about filmmaking either. Walking into the room of a family that has money, or a family that's a big family with a lot of support, you see the balloons, you see the flowers, the laptops, the game boys, the teddy bears, the special blankets and pillows, the letters from their school, pictures on the wall. But in kids' rooms whose parents are strapped financially, there is generally very little of that.

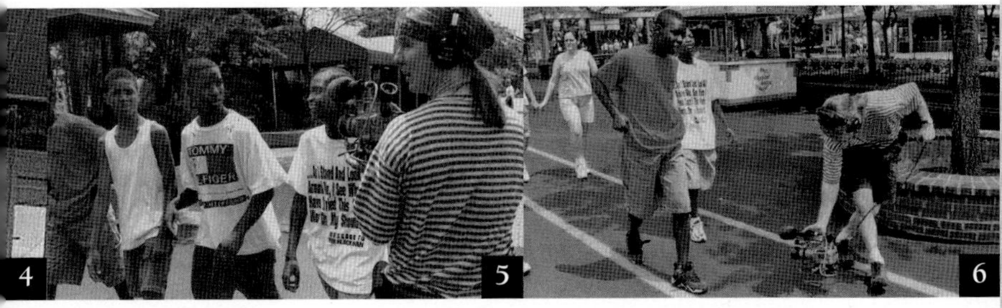

1. Steve filming Al Fields in the early days.

2. Steve films surgery.

3. Julia films surgery.

4. Julia being interviewed by Al Fields. "How do you like filming?" was his first question. Al loved the camera.

5. Steve films Tim and his cousins, Greg and Roy, and friend Tony, at the King's Island Amusement Park, on a trip with Tim's nurse Connie, and her husband, Rob.

6. Close up of the moving feet. Steve has a unique shooting style.

We kept in touch with the hospital and the families as best we could. But we also had other responsibilities, including our day jobs. Keeping up with five families isn't so easy—they're busy folks, we're busy folks, and good intentions don't always lead you to pick up the phone. Yet for a documentarian, the moments you miss are the moments you remember. We missed a big chapter in Jen's story. It was very dramatic, and a great example of how for a kid fighting cancer, there's danger everywhere. Jen and her family, like pretty much every kid fighting cancer, were given a "Special Wish." They chose a trip to Disneyworld. Well, while at Disneyworld, they ate at a restaurant, and they all got food poisoning. For the rest of the family, this meant an uncomfortable day. But for Jen, a kid with no immune system, this could be completely life threatening. And poor Jen spent the next two weeks in the hospital, fighting for her life. Well, unfortunately, we missed the whole thing.

Editing and Post Production

STEVEN:

Julia and I and our editing colleagues have struggled pretty much every week for the nearly five years it took to edit this film, with how to tell this story, how to do right by these families, while still telling the truth.

And in a way, you could say, that's the documentarian's job: to do right by the truth, while doing right by the people who trusted you. And to tell a good story. But the question of trust and trustworthiness comes up again and again.

My journey in making this film led to a threshold I finally crossed, where I would not put the camera down as things got too intimate or intense.

When we started shooting, at first I was so skittish about staying in people's rooms too long, or asking them difficult questions. Julia always had tougher or braver instincts than me.

Someone once asked me if I had ice water in my veins to film some of the stuff we filmed. That comment hurt, because I believe an essential part of being a true documentarian is that you film hard stuff and somehow keep the ice water away. You film hard stuff and you let yourself feel it, keeping your humanity open to the pain of the situation you are filming. This isn't easy, it keeps your heart ripped open, and it can damage you if you're not careful. But it is a necessary element of being an ethical documentarian.

A few months later, we filmed the moment when Tim and Marietha are told the news that Tim's cancer had come back. I happened to be shooting that day, and as usual the camera

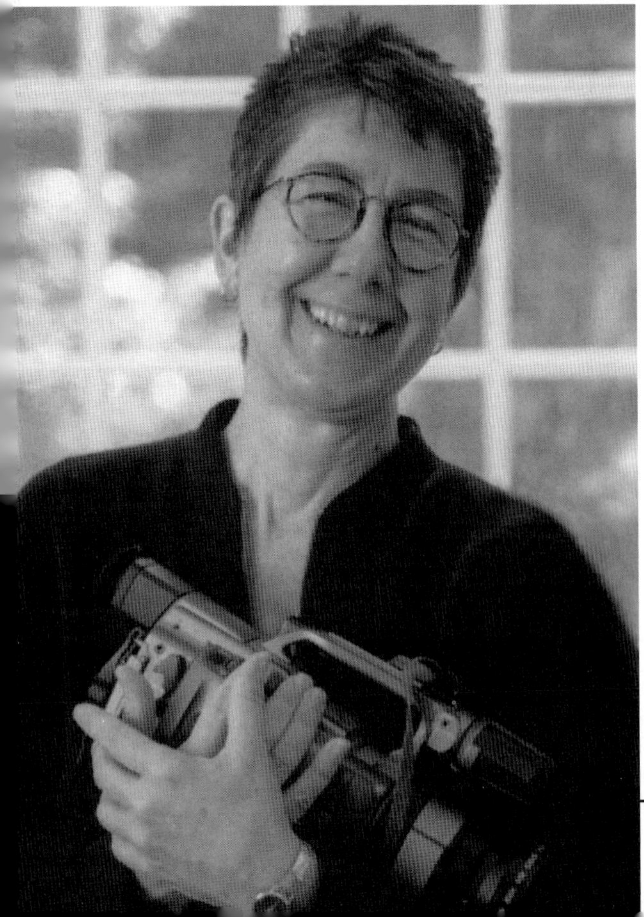

Julia and her video camera, in her studio at the MacDowell Colony.

was very close to Tim (our backs were snug against the wall of the small hospital room).

As his doctors tell the news, Tim starts crying. He's only two feet away and he's crying because he just found out his cancer's coming back. And I'm holding a lens on him. A voice in my head said, "Put that damn camera down, you asshole, and comfort him." But I didn't put the camera down, and Julia did not put the boom pole down.

We looked at this amazing young man, we offered what sympathy we could with our eyes, with brief words. But we kept shooting.

I felt so ashamed of myself afterwards—I felt I had not done right by him or his dignity. Julia and I talked about it a lot on the long car ride home, and in the weeks that followed. We told ourselves we weren't obliged to use that footage. Or we could trim it way down, in the editing. Yeah, right. Here was a deeply powerful scene and we're trying to kid ourselves into thinking we won't use it.

A few years later, when we first went to a documentary festival in Toronto called Hot Docs, I got a chance to see Christian Frei's great documentary *War Photographer*, about photojournalist James Nachtwey. In the film, you see Nachtwey shooting pictures in some of the most difficult circumstances on earth, where moms, dads and kids are suffering profoundly. Nachtwey expresses hope that his photos will make a difference, and yet, to my surprise, he also talks about the shame he feels at times.

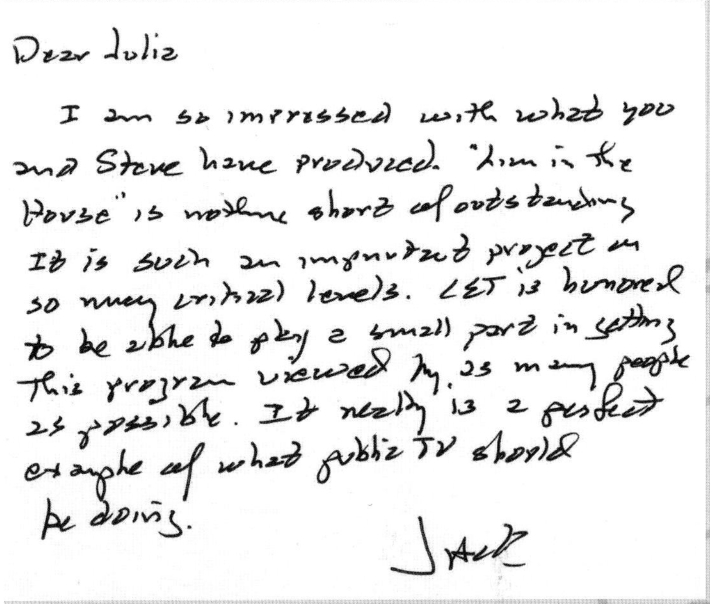
Dear Julia

I am so impressed with what you and Steve have produced. "Lion in the House" is nothing short of outstanding. It is such an important project on so many critical levels. CET is honored to be able to play a small part in getting this program viewed by as many people as possible. It really is a perfect example of what public TV should be doing.

Jack

This card, from PBS station CET in Cincinnati, gave us early support, years ago.
Dear Julia,
I am so impressed with what you and Steve produced. Lion in the House *is nothing short of outstanding. It is such an important project on so many critical levels. CET is honored to be able to play a small part in getting this program viewed by as many people as possible. It really is a perfect example of what public TV should be doing.*
Jack (Dominic)

Hearing this made a huge difference to me—to know that shame is a part of this job, a necessary check in the process of doing ethical work. Julia has a very different view of this complicated subject. But Nachtwey's (and Frei's) words allowed me to make a crucial shift; you can feel shame and yet still do the right thing in filming. The shame should be there, as a measure of your conscience.

The terrifying nuns at my Catholic schools would say no, that the ends do not justify the means. But you make a pact. Both parties in a documentary, the looker and the looked-at, make a pact to tell the truth. And if both parties hold to that pact, then you can't put your camera down. If Tim didn't tell me to put the camera down, I wouldn't. Is that a dubious justification? Some would say yes. But that kind of ground rule is also how good documentaries get made.

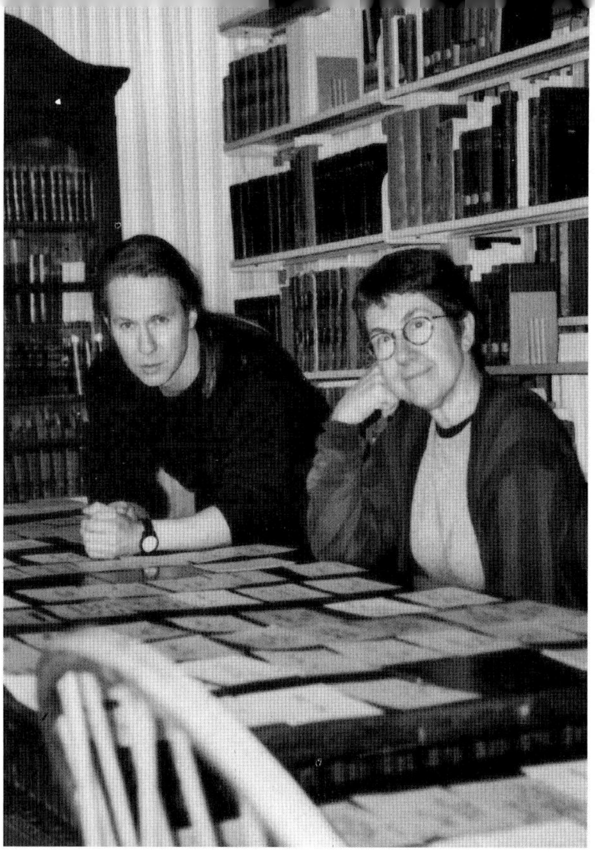

Steve and Julia working at the Antioch College library.
"A lot of our editing happened on cards and in our minds. Each scene had an index card. Each family had a different color card. Here we are trying to figure out the narrative structure of the film by moving the cards around."

JULIA:

Shame never entered into my mind. This was my view: the families agreed we should be there, and document, no matter what. It was our job. Our primary reason to be there was not as a caregiver, not as a friend, though we were those somewhat.

We were there to be witness, to document, and then to take on the responsibility of sharing that with the world. That meant to keep shooting unless the families asked us to stop.

To me, if we put the camera down at hard times, we would not be doing our job. It really helped clarify for me how to be in those moments. It took a while to figure this out, that we had taken on this job and we had damn well better do the best we could.

We were privileged to be witness to some extraordinary human interactions. Witnessing for us meant documenting. That was our job. Witnessing also meant going the next step: dedication to getting the film out to millions of people, working to be sure the film was as useful as possible. It meant being honest witness to all the events and to all the sides, all the perspectives that were part of the things we were observing. And I don't believe I ever felt a second of shame.

STEVEN:

Once we had taped over a hundred hours of footage, we realized that keeping it organized would be a major challenge. I developed a few systems, like quick reference charts, and Julia took on the huge job of getting all the footage logged, transcribed. Because at the rate we were filming, we knew that if it wasn't all thoroughly logged, we'd never know what tape contained this visit, or that meeting, or the moment when someone said something great.

JULIA:

Logging over 500 hours of tape was a big job. At first, our interns from Antioch College, and former students of mine from Wright State University's film program, helped out. But the sheer volume of work made it slow going. And not everyone has the aptitude for logging. For a while, Dave Ackels, our friend, my former student, and an excellent documentary filmmaker, volunteered to log. But he got so frustrated with it that he hand-wrote notes in the margins. Things like, "This is so boring," and, "Steve, I'm going to kick your ass if you keep filming everything." I ran into a friend of ours, Mary T. White, who I knew to be on the faculty at the Wright State School of Medicine. Mary also lives in Yellow Springs, and like many projects that start in this town, our collaboration began in the local grocery store. I ran into her and invited her over to our house to see some scenes from the rough cut with a few other people. When it was over, Mary said, "I want to use this in class tomorrow." Turns out Mary is a "medical ethicist"—that's what she teaches.

Before too long we came in and showed a short clip of the film to a med school class. It seemed to really engage the students. Afterwards, I mentioned to Mary the difficulty in getting all the footage logged, and she suggested we see if any of the WSU School of Medicine students would be interested in helping out. Mary said they may be able to receive a kind of credit, for community service, by helping us out. What we didn't fully anticipate was how engaged in much of the process these students would become. They found it instructive to see the much longer raw footage from the film.

Their engagement made a huge difference in getting the work done. A few of the students, who are all doctors now, by the way, really went the extra mile, including Rebecca Podurgiel, Rama Chandrashekaran and Kate Conway. The School of Medicine eventually appointed me a Professor of Community Health, and it's been very meaningful to me to see these students, who helped us, at their graduation and hooding ceremony, where they are first named doctors.

STEVEN:

A good example of how we approached editing the difficult scenes in the film is Jen's spinal tap. In the final film, this scene is 30 to 40 seconds long. In real life, it was at least 20 minutes, if not

Julia and Steve at the graduation of Dr. Rebecca Podiergel from the Wright State University School of Medicine. Rebecca and other classmates at the WSU Medical School, over several years, did the vast bulk of logging and transcribing the footage from A Lion in the House.

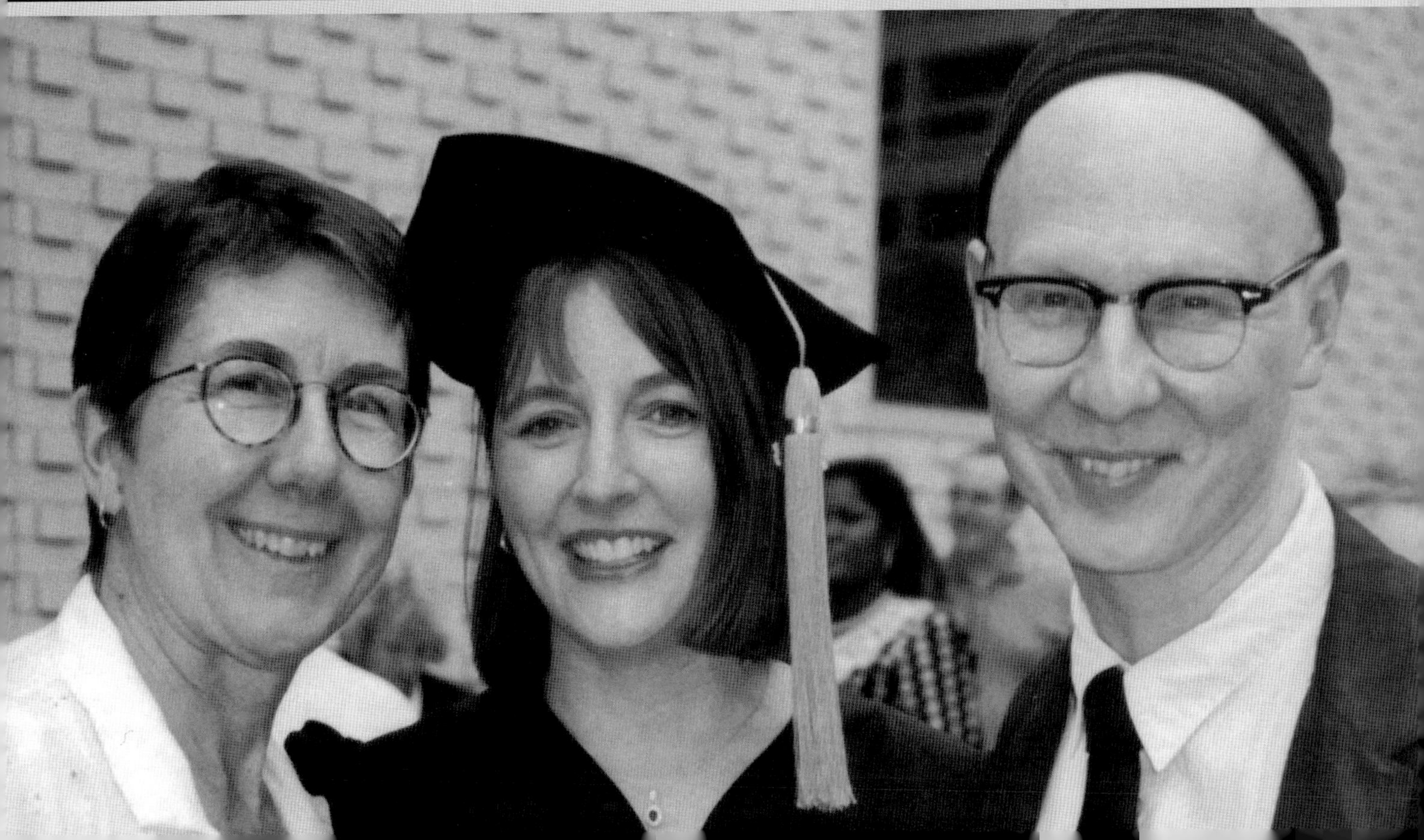

half an hour. They actually had to go in twice that day, two needles. So when we first cut the scene together, it was something like 6 or 7 minutes long. We thought we had already cut it way down, from real time.

JULIA:

But when we started showing it, our small test audiences—meaning our friends and neighbors—couldn't handle it. One dear friend nearly fainted. And later, one of my students actually did faint during a test screening. In my memory, I can still hear the clunk of his head hitting a desk!

STEVEN:

So for almost four years, that scene gradually got shorter and shorter, little by little, until audiences didn't emotionally, emphatically say to us, "It's too long!" But see, we never wanted to betray the power of the scene by making it too short. That would not honor Jen's courage. Yet it had to be watchable. We couldn't have people fainting. So specific decisions, like how long each shot lasts, how long do we stay on the close-up of the scary needle. All this was gradually and organically figured out.

JULIA:

But editing wore on our souls. It certainly wore on Steve's soul. It wore on my soul differently, in that I knew the thing we were trying to put together was absolutely enormous, and an enormous responsibility, and, were we up for the task? Month after month of cutting, of seeing that things were still wrong, and how far we had to go. He bore the lion's share of that.

I think the outreach wore on my soul, more than on Steve's. I always felt like we were never doing enough.

I thought it took a terrible toll on Steve, in the editing. And that was painful to me. A fair amount of the drive to get other editors here was my doing. It was always risky, because they might not have been right, or good. They might have been trouble. But I could see the damage being done to Steve. And yet there was nothing else to be done but keep going.

STEVEN:

It's not easy for me to describe how hard the editing process was. It's like first we had been through an amazing and profoundly challenging experience, in filming these stories and

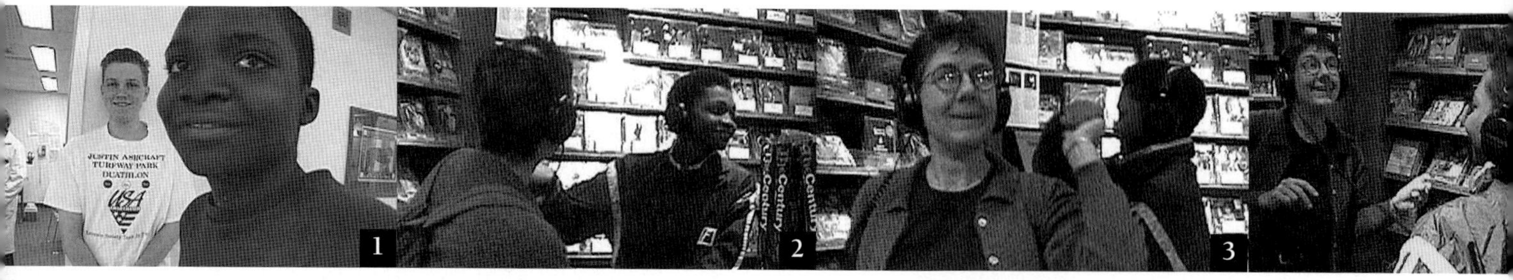

spending all that time with the families. And the experience of losing the kids we lost—going through the deaths of Justin, Alex and Tim—this was the hardest thing I'd ever been through in my life, up to then. And they weren't even our kids. That's what makes me realize how unimaginable it is, for anyone who hasn't been through it, to know what it is to lose a child, how unimaginable that pain must be. Because even though we had only known these kids for a short part of their life, their deaths were deeply, deeply painful. I went into a fairly long period of depression after they died. So with that as the prologue, we began editing the film, and reliving these deeply painful moments again and again and again. For years. Looking at these kids suffering again and again, day in and day out, reliving their deaths and funerals, week after week, month after month. It was hard. Profoundly hard. At the same time, I would not have traded it for anything, because this was, this is, the responsibility that came to us. It was our job, our mission, to tell these stories. But I've now watched and listened to these deeply painful scenes I don't know how many times. Hundreds. The pictures and sounds stay in my mind. It's taken a psychic toll. With the movie done and able to stand on its own, I'm hoping I don't have to watch these scenes again.

I know I'm not the same person I was when we started this film. I've seen too much trouble and pain, too much sorrow and death. But I've also seen the full capacity of the human heart, and the full measure of love, and these are gifts that have expanded me as a person. These are gifts I use every day.

The Fellowship of the Lion

JULIA:

We put together a kick-ass editing team. Our first consulting editor, who is also one of the film's final editors, is Jim Klein. Jim's sought after by filmmakers around the country as an editor and consulting editor. We're so lucky he lives in our town. He's also the father of Lela, and my former partner, and my friend of almost forty years. He's been woven into the fabric of making this film since it began. We had young kids at first, to help us rough cut scenes together from raw footage. They included Kevin Jones, Jaime Meyers, Sarah Silver, Brent Huffman, Beth O'Brien, Leilah Weinraub and Peter Ridgeway. It was valuable experience for new, emerging filmmakers, and it helped us a ton in taking the 525 hours of raw footage down to a watchable first cut, which was something like twenty-eight hours long. This film wouldn't be what it is without our creative collaborators.

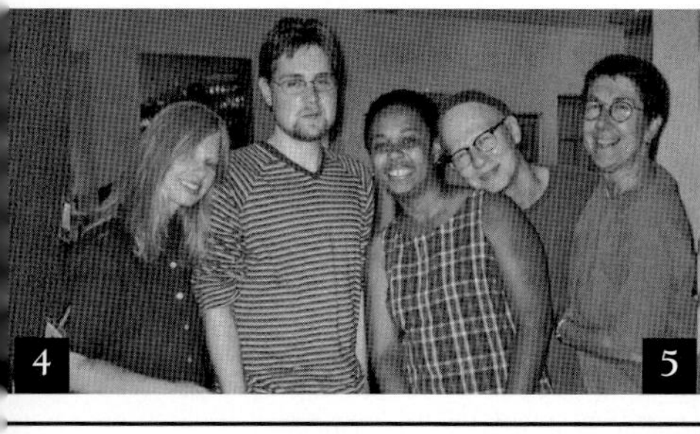
4

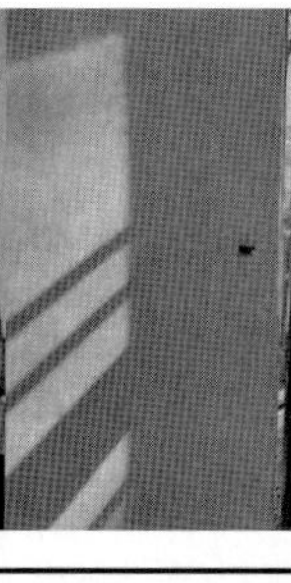
5

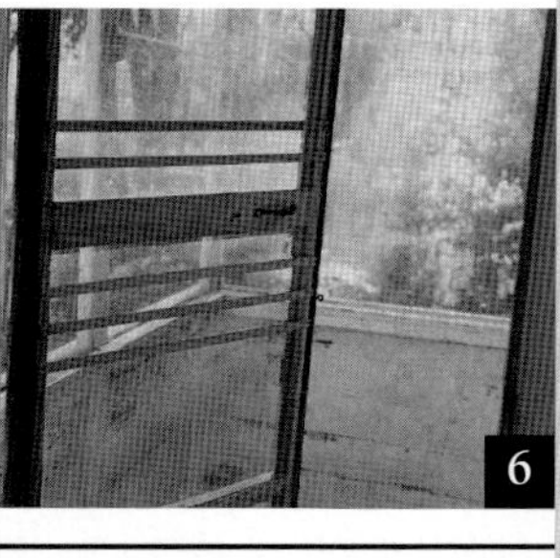
6

1. Justin and Tim meet in the hallway at Cincinnati Children's.

2-4. Julia and Tim dancing in a record store in Chicago.

5. Editors Jaime Meyers and Brent Huffman and award winning filmmaker and LION consultant Selena Burks with Steve and Julia.

6. Bungalow view.

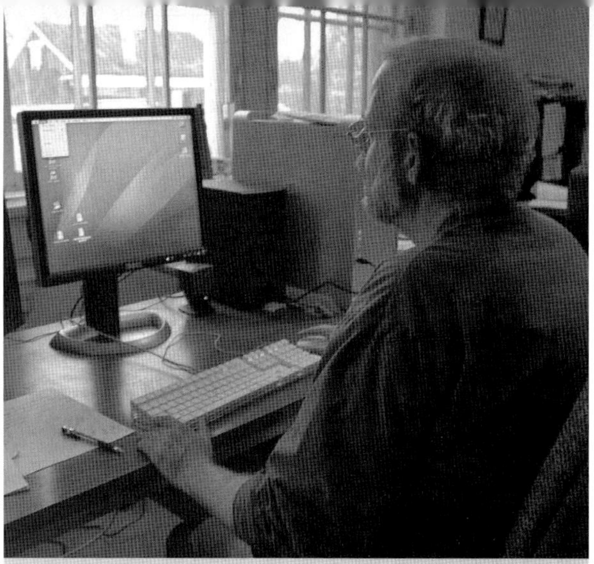

Jim Klein, senior consulting editor, at work in the finishing stages of Lion.

STEVEN:

It was an organic process, of finding this team. Kind of like the poor farmers in *Seven Samurai*, who wander the countryside looking for the small band of warriors who can defend their village. In general, we are always assessing people's talents and interest and level of passion. The two of us talk about the people we meet, to see if we could ever work with them. The fact that Julia teaches at the acclaimed film school at Wright State University gives her concrete knowledge of who in that community is a hard worker, who has editing ability, who has personal standards of excellence.

The final *Lion* editing team included Kevin Jones, Mary Lampson, Jim Klein, Jaime Meyers as senior editors, Ann Rotolante and Sarah Silver as associate editors and Brent Huffman, Leilah Weinraub, Beth O'Brien and Peter Ridgeway as assistant editors. They all really let the material get under their skin, into their hearts. That matters a lot with this film. Beyond the editors, our producing colleagues, like Karen Durgans and Melissa Godoy, looked at much material and gave their valuable feedback, again and again.

JULIA:

These editors came up with crucial ideas, like the gradual realization we had that the film shouldn't start with Jen Moone and Al Fields, because their stories get spread too thin if they span the entire four hours. So even though for years, literally years, the movie began with Al and Jen, now we were looking for a new direction. Kevin Jones, one of the senior editors on the film, came up with the major idea that Jen and Al should begin part 2, to bring in fresh energy, and to start part 2 in a way that distinguishes itself from part 1.

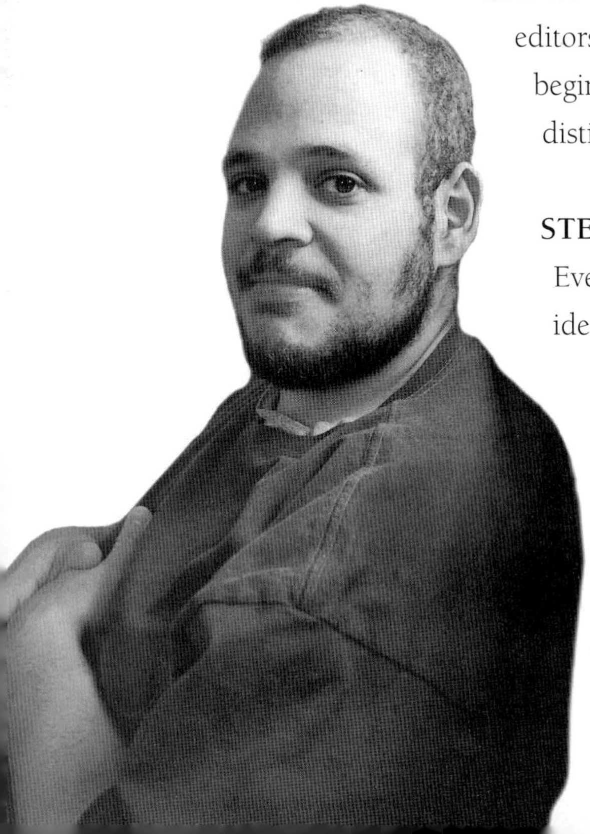

STEVEN:

Every editor on this film contributed big ideas, structurally, tone-wise, idea-wise. Kevin also deserves real credit for finally figuring out how to end the movie. For the longest time, the movie had a way too long series of endings, scene after scene of the families moving forward in time, gradually doing better. We were in love with many of these small scenes and moments, and we were having difficulty letting go of them. Kevin took what was something like a 20-minute, maybe 25-minute sequence and took it down

Editor Kevin Jones also began early on, then moved to Northern California. But he was persuaded to move back to small-town Ohio several times to help with the final editing.

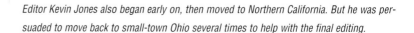

to something like 7 minutes. In doing this, he created a "coda" which was a more visual experience—more cinematic. He found the essence of each family's ending story, and he wove it together masterfully. The first time we watched it, with consulting editors Austin Allen and Michelle Davis, we all just cried our eyes out.

JULIA:

The consulting editors were crucial. We knew a lot about the film, but there was still a lot to learn.

One good thing about the American documentary community is we generally find the time to watch each other's cuts, give each other honest notes, help each other out. These are people who love the craft as much as we do. We have certain people we turn to, and we enlarged the circle with this big project. Friends and colleagues from past projects, like Yvonne Welbon, Gordon Quinn, Tony Heriza, Erik Bork and Russ Johnson. New compatriots, like Rob Moss, Steve James, David Simpson and Brad Lichtenstein.

ITVS connected us to Nathaniel Dorsky, who is a noted experimental filmmaker by day, but who also works as an amazing consulting editor on documentary projects. Nathaniel, who goes by Nick, offered wisdom like a kung fu master—these short koans of editing wisdom. "You must switch your allegiance from the material to the film." "Let's not be mediocre just because we're in trouble," and, "Don't second-guess it into the shithouse."

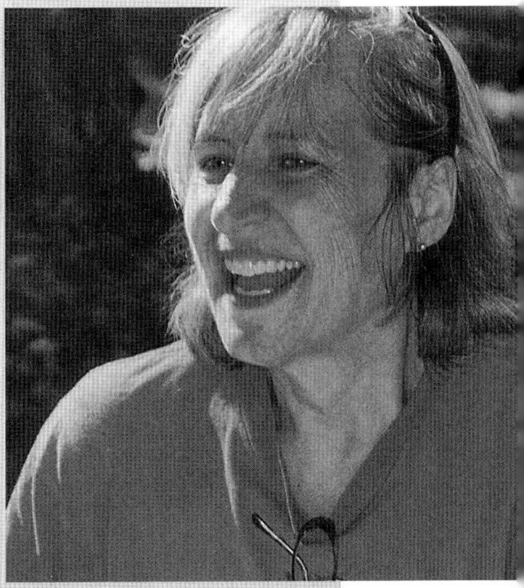

Editor Mary Lampson, who moved to Ohio for nearly a year to contribute greatly to the Lion *edit.*

MARY LAMPSON, Editor:

I actually had breast cancer myself, so for me working on the film wasn't entering the world of cancer. I had been there already.

Before I got sick, when I went to the pediatrician's office with my kids, I would walk up these three stairs where the sign to the right pointed to pediatrics, and to the left to the main center for cancer and blood disorders. I remember seeing that sign and thinking, "Thank God I don't have to turn left."

Then the day came when I had to turn left. I had to walk down that hall and open that door and enter a world nobody wants to go into. But I did and it's an amazing world.

For me what the film does is bring the audience into that place. In an amazing way, it says to the audience, "You will be taken care of while we take you to this horrible place. You're going to be changed by the experience."

Anybody who has had cancer and gone into that world has had that experience. It's a scary world, but it's an extraordinary world. You find out things about yourself and the people who love you and the people who take care of you in many, many amazing ways.

After having cancer, I had this feeling I had been changed in a way that's hard to articulate.

Nobody could understand who hadn't been through it themselves. I wanted to do something to express some of those things through my work, to communicate to other people the power of what it had done to me. In many ways I feel that horrible experience made me a better person. It sounds really corny, but it made me wiser and stronger and funnier and less afraid and all these very deep things.

I have known Julia since the '70s, but fate brought me to their film. I had been out of the filmmaker world for a long time, and had just decided to get back into it, so I went to New York to renew contacts.

I was walking through Union Square after I came out of the subway and said to myself, "Wouldn't it be funny if I bumped into Marc Weiss?" I looked up and there was Marc Weiss. He was a close friend of Julia's and mine from the late '60s/early 70's. We go way back. He said, "What are you doing?" I said, "I'm just getting back into editing." This is after twenty-two years of living in Maine. He said, "I'm going to a birthday party Julia is throwing for Steve. Why don't you go with me?" I couldn't, but he went, and Julia said, "We're looking for an editor," and Marc said, "I just bumped into Mary," and that's how I ended up working on the film.

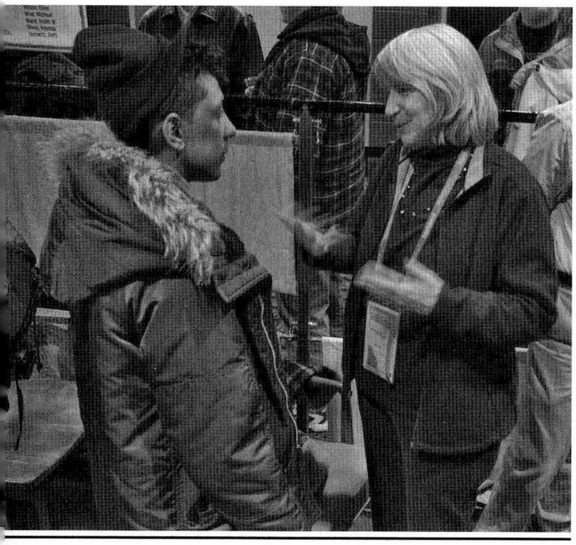

Even though they both worked hard on the film, Editor Mary Lampson and Assistant Editor Leilah Weinraub meet for the first time at Sundance. Given that the film took nearly five years to edit, most of the editing team did not work concurrently on the film.

I think that's just an incredible story. That's fate. There's no way Julia would have known I was back. There's no way I would have known they were looking for help.

I went to Ohio for eight months to work on the film. I worked on the middle part of it. It was at 13 or 14 hours long when I started working with them to bring it down to about seven hours. The hard thing about that kind of movie is not to feel you're invading people's privacy somewhere. What I found extraordinary was the clear relationship Julia and Steve established with everybody they had come into contact with. It wasn't at all a voyeuristic thing. What you are doing is bearing witness. The film brings the audience in and says, "We know this will be very, very hard, but you are safe with us." That was the challenge, to make the audience feel that way. It was a profound.

JAIME MEYERS, Editor:

When I started working as an editor for *A Lion in the House*, I had no idea the impact it would have on my life.

Filmmaking is a collaborative art. But working with the *Lion* team felt like being part of a family, with a common goal driving us, to be respectful of people who allowed us to witness some of the most intimate parts of their lives, who trusted us to craft their story with a careful hand.

We spent days editing, and then watching the scenes we had put together. There were constant discussions about what was most important to tell. The collaboration was invaluable.

It was during this documentary that I truly fell in love with the process of editing. It became a

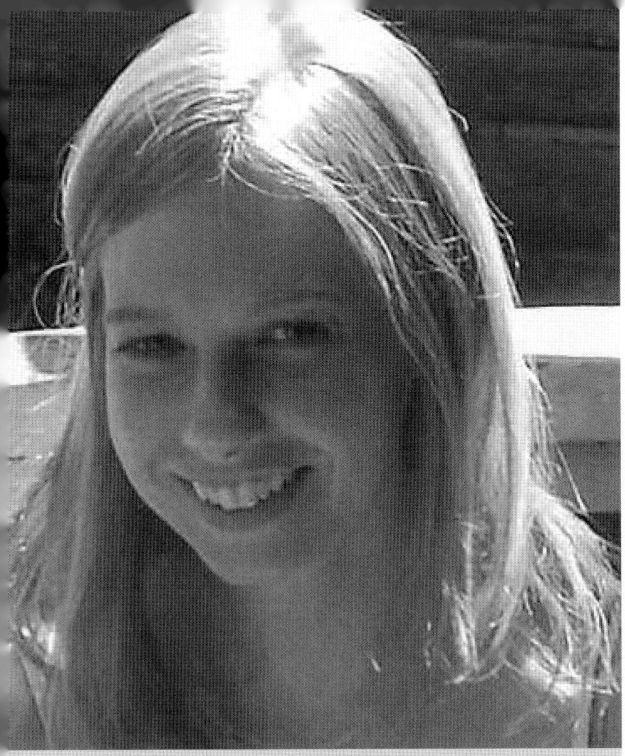

Jaime Meyers was one of the first editors on the film.

joy to go through hours and hours of footage and find the little moments that stand out, that people remember, that make up lives. It's where I learned the difference between just working on a project, and working on something that my heart was into. Knowing this difference has stayed with me.

I will always remember the bungalow, which is what we called the small apartment in Yellow Springs that Steve and Julia turned into an editing suite, where we all spent so many hours. I'll remember the strange way the silence would be broken by the hum of the computers as so many hard drives booted up. The balcony was nice to sit on, especially when it was raining, when I needed a moment to allow the footage I'd seen that day to sink in.

I felt connected with the families in the documentary, even though I had never met them. When I saw footage of Al feeling well and playing basketball, I was happy. When I watched Justin's mom, Debbie, see her son for the first time after brain surgery, I cried. When I finally got a chance to meet some of the families, all I could do was hug them, and thank them.

The people who were a part of *A Lion in the House,* both in the film and around it, will always have a special place in my heart and mind. I will always be thankful for the experience, and be honored to have been a part of it.

MELISSA GODOY, Line Producer:

To me, working on *Lion* has been a dream come true. A privilege. To work on a film that I care about a lot, with people who care as much. I don't mind the long hours. This is my life. There is no line between who I am and what I'm working on. Everybody on this crew is the same way. Even more encouraging is Steve and Julia's constant pursuit of excellence, never, ever satisfied with "good enough." Their complete openness—no, not openness—that's an understatement. Their active solicitation of criticism to make the film constantly better is remarkable and courageous. It makes me giggle when I think about editors who complain about a 2nd or 3rd revision. I witnessed this group of artists revise endlessly, obsessively, as a team. All with the same goal: to move people in the tiniest moments. To harness emotion and shape, to tell the story in the subtlest of ways. It is also amazing that Steve and Julia built in so much time to experiment, to shift scene orders, add and subtract shots, and test the

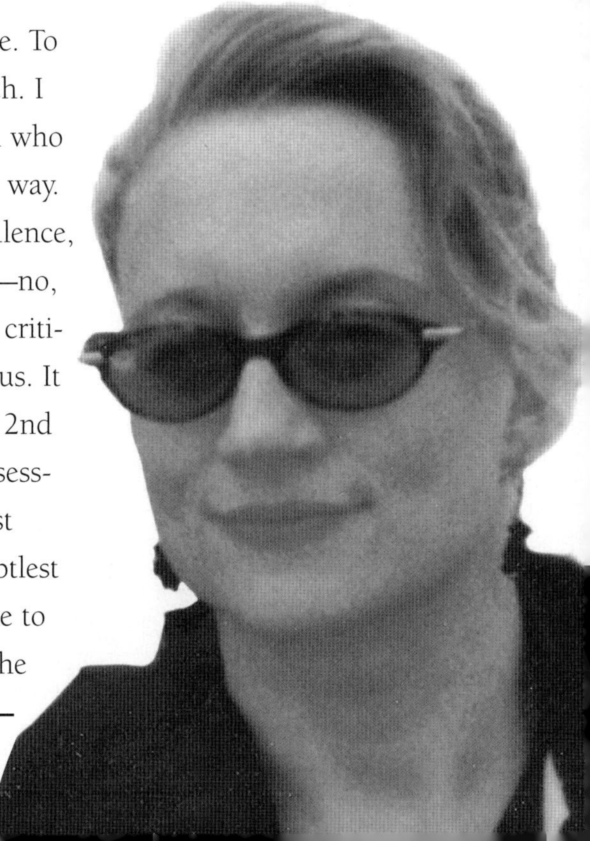

Line Producer Melissa Godoy

effects on an audience. For Steve and Julia, this part of the process is a must and the results show. They learned what makes an audience care about these characters or when the audience becomes weary. They learned how to build investment in the story and to tell truth that is as compelling as fiction.

I might add that the relentless drive for excellence extends to every aspect of the film, from outreach to you-name-it. No stone goes unturned.

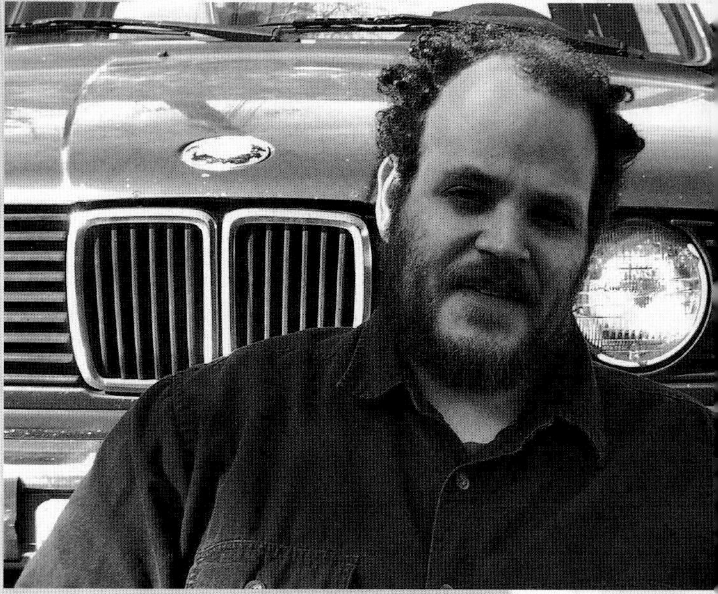

Kevin Jones AKA King Jones.

There are two parts of the film that get me the most. The first is when Alex goes home for the last time and she cries because she is happy. She receives a tender farewell by Dr. Arceci and the nurse. Then she is wheeled off in the loving care of her family. It is in that moment I sense a higher power.

The other moment is when Marietha sits by Tim's hospital bed sobbing as her wide-eyed, terrified and brilliant son fights for his life.

This moment almost always sparks a parallel reflection in my mind about how she labored to bring him into this world only sixteen years earlier. She herself only eighteen, in another hospital bed. How unprepared she was when she had to "give him back."

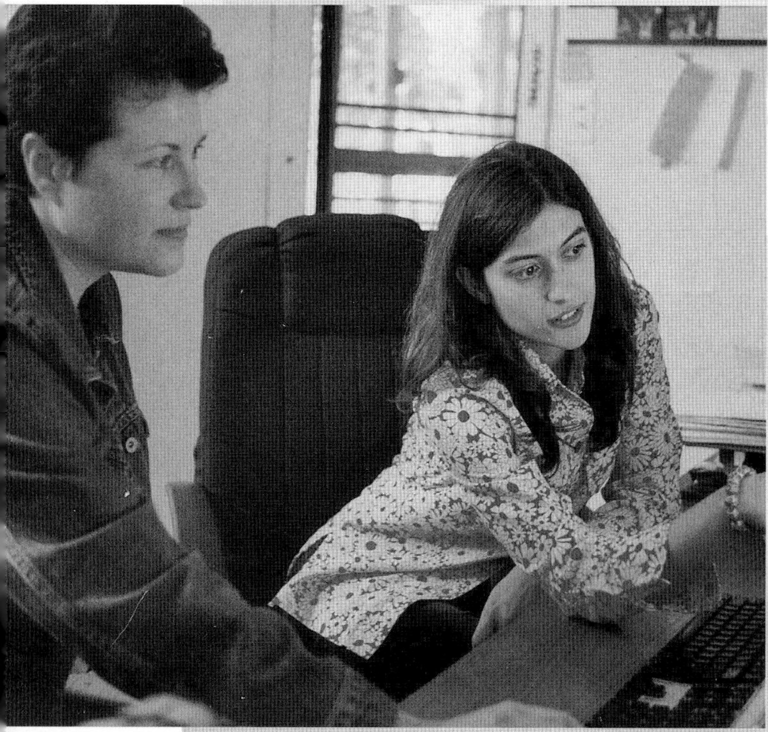

Anne Rotolante and Sarah Silver working in the bungalow.

ANNE ROTOLANTE, Associate Editor, Post-Production "Superwoman":

I've always thought of editors as "guns for hire." We walk into a project with no emotional connection to the material, surgically shape it through the brutal act of cutting, then leave when our job is done, unscathed. While this has been my experience with other films I've edited, in the case of *A Lion in the House* nothing could be further from the truth.

Among Wright State University "Mopix" (motion picture production) students and alumni, Julia and Steve's "cancer doc" is legend. Perhaps because it has been in production and editing for so long, perhaps because so many of us have worked on it over the years, no one believed that it might actually be nearing completion. Julia approached me in mid-2005 to help out a few days a week as a part-timer because Steve needed help getting the project completed. Back in July 2003 I had worked for a week on *A Lion in the House* as an assistant editor. I was familiar with some of the material and would only be on the project for that last final push; it sounded easy enough, so I signed on.

My first assignment was to look at a recent cut of the film. It had been cut from something like sixty hours to six and a half. I was able to maintain a cool professional distance from the material for the first hour or so of the program. But before I realized what was happening, I found myself being drawn in. Each child and each family had such an interesting story, and it was so easy to become emotionally invested in them. As the film progressed, it was heartbreaking to learn that not every child survived. And then I wanted to know what happened next to the families, and to the children who did survive. How did their lives turn out? Had they moved on? Would cancer cast a shadow over them forever? I just fell into the film like any viewer.

Then Steve delivered the news that we would be taking the six and a half hour cut of the film down to four hours. Kevin Jones was spearheading the cut. Kevin did an amazing job of getting us on the right path before he left the project in July 2005. But there was still a minute here and there that we had to trim to get the film to the right running time for PBS. What scenes could we lose? Every moment seemed so right, and to lose anything would change the flow of the film and the emotional tone of each child's story. Julia and Steve agonized over these decisions. As work continued, my part-time status evolved into full-time plus, with work bleeding over into nights and weekends.

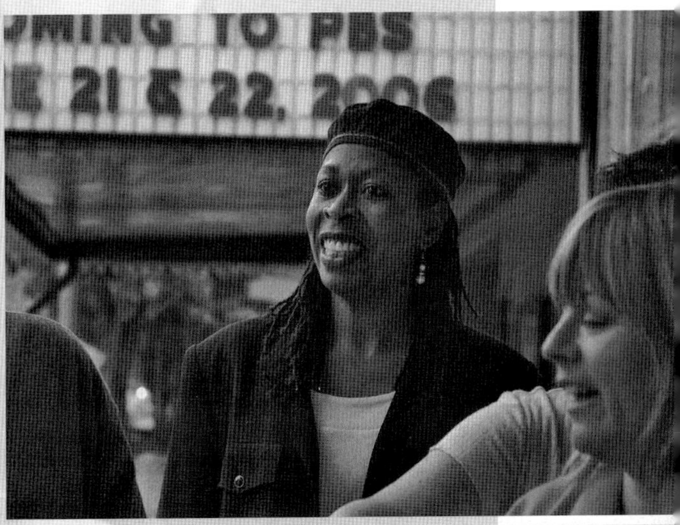

Karen Durgans

KAREN DURGANS, Outreach Coordinator:

From the first week that I met Julia and Steve in November of 2002, they talked about outreach. They didn't want *Lion*, then a still loosely shaped documentary, to air one day and be gone the next without making a lasting impact. I learned about Lela being a survivor of childhood cancer, and over time I learned just how much Lela, and the five kids, their families, the doctors and nurses had so deeply affected Steve and Julia, especially those who were dealing with economic and social disparities.

STEVEN:

Julia poured her heart and soul into the outreach efforts. Relatively early on, she found great colleagues in Jim Sommers and Susan Latton of ITVS. They all saw the potential of this film, the need to choose specific content areas, and the ball got rolling.

KAREN:

This focus on outreach drew my attention right away and I felt I had a place with Julia and Steve because of my background as a licensed professional counselor and years of doing social work in the Cincinnati area where *Lion* was filmed. My Mom and her two sisters are breast cancer survivors. I have had two scares—lumps in my breasts—so addressing cancer was also personally compelling. Also, I had just completed an intense, documentary program offered through a unique relationship between Suffolk University's Business School and the producers of a public television series called *Visionaries*.

After graduation from Suffolk's Visionaries Institute, I came back to Yellow Springs not knowing about Julia, Steve, or *A Lion in the House*. Julia had placed an ad in the local newspaper that busy filmmakers needed an office manager; I applied and was accepted. The second week I was there, Julia and Steve left for six weeks to edit the film in New York and to begin meeting with national leaders of key organizations who dealt with cancer or cancer-related issues.

Since I was working in their home, I was amazed that this couple trusted me to come and go, without really knowing me. I came to understand that knowing how and when to extend trust, and to do so generously, is an endearing part of their make-up.

Steve and Julia on the path to their artist studios, on the wooded acres of the MacDowell Colony, outside of Peterborough, New Hampshire. MacDowell has been a creative haven for artists over the last century. Says Julia, "Our film would not go as deep if we had not gone to MacDowell."

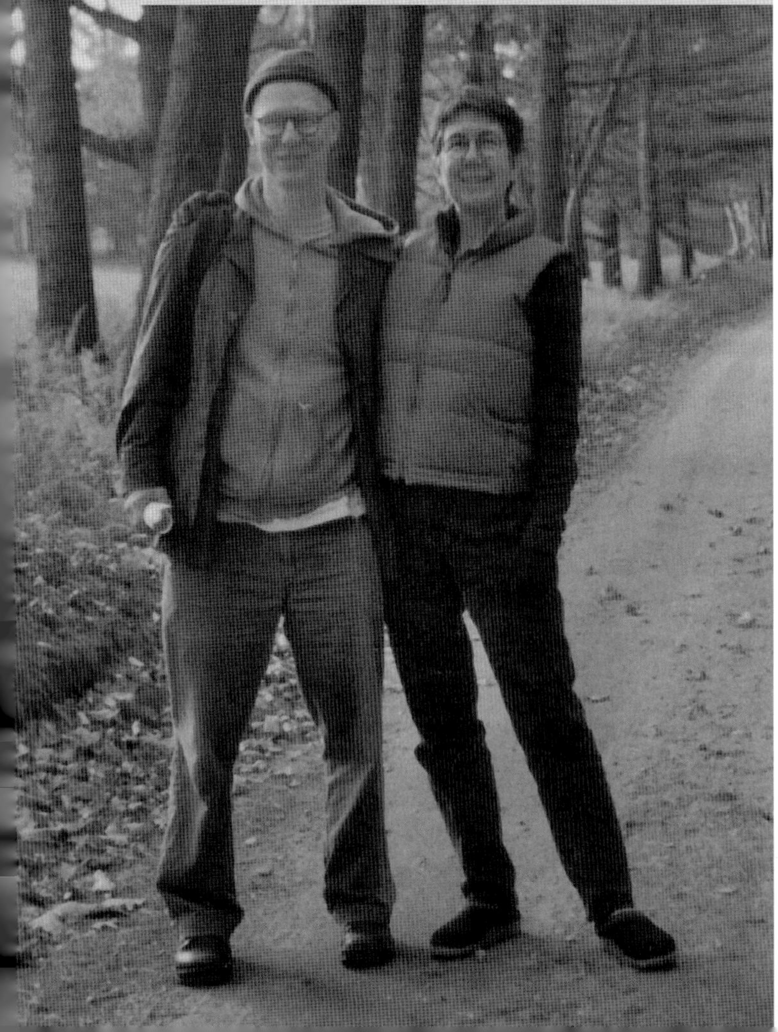

JULIA:

Between 2001 and 2005, we did many test screenings of the rough cuts, mostly in our living room. We're so very fortunate to have friends and neighbors willing to spend a lot of time—entire weekends, at times—watching full cuts of the film and giving us extensive feedback. We also did these at ITVS and the MacDowell Colony, and the feedback was crucial. We developed questionnaires, had long discussions and served meals as needed.

KAREN:

Many students and staff became personal friends with Julia and Steve, and/or entered the local filmmaking community, often working on other projects together. The screenings provided another opportunity for Julia and Steve to reach out to the community at large, inviting trusted friends and colleagues, and recommending sages of all ages, races, and walks of life to provide valued and seriously considered input. Steve and

Julia kneaded this mix with professional film doctors who guided them to skillfully allow the stories to emerge and to choose only the best of the best scenes to tell the story. I was in awe of the humility of the filmmakers and their interdependence with community. I wanted to be like that when I grow up.

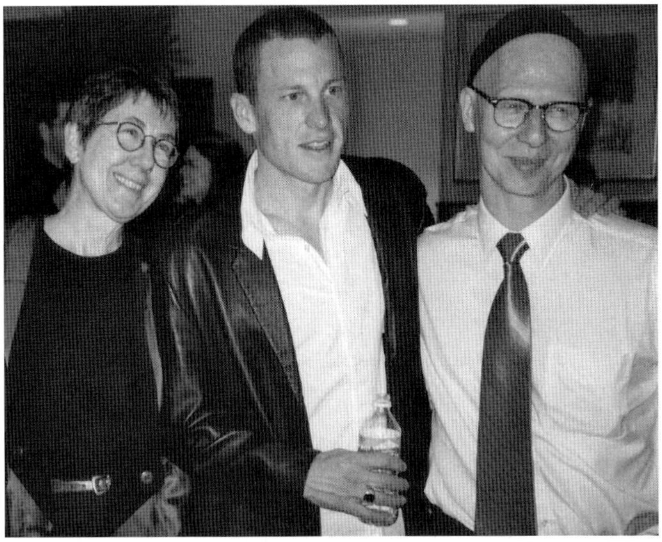

Julia, Lance Armstrong and Steve at a fundraising event for the Starbright Foundation and the Lance Armstrong Foundation in Los Angeles. The support of the LAF has been strong and steady for Lion *since they discovered the film at the rough cut stage.*

Outreach flourished exponentially. Jim Sommers, then director of outreach at ITVS, recruited Susan Latton, national outreach consultant, to help lead the effort. Jim and Susan participated in the first regional outreach summit in Cincinnati, then, launched their efforts to recruit national partners. ITVS and the Lance Armstrong Foundation awarded grants of $10,000 to 10 PBS stations across the country for outreach projects, with CET (Cincinnati Educational Television—the PBS affiliate) in Cincinnati being one of the winners.

Julia and Steve presented early on to 1,200 people at the Intercultural Cancer Council's Ninth Biennial Symposium on Cancer, Minorities, and the Medically Underserved. Julia presented to C-Change, which includes the President's Cancer Panel, and to the Children's Oncology Group, the group that sets the protocols for hospitals that treat 90 percent of children fighting cancer. Julia and Steve received a grant from the Centers of Disease Control and Prevention, the first ever between a public television venture and the CDC, to alert young adult survivors of childhood cancer of their risks for late effects from their cancer treatment.

JULIA:

The "Survivor Alert" project (www.survivoralert.org) is close to my heart, because of my kid Lela, because of the kids in the film, and because of the young adult survivors I've known, some of whom are doing fine, some of whom have late side effects of their treatment. It will mean a lot to me if this project can empower young adults who've survived cancer to take charge of their life and long-term health.

Sundance and surprises

ANNE:

For a long time, I thought that the hardest part of working on *A Lion in the House* would be making sure that we were all happy with the four-hour cut. At times we felt like the film had lost its guts and soul and we had to find it again.

Then as we approached our deadline for sound mix and color correction, I thought that would

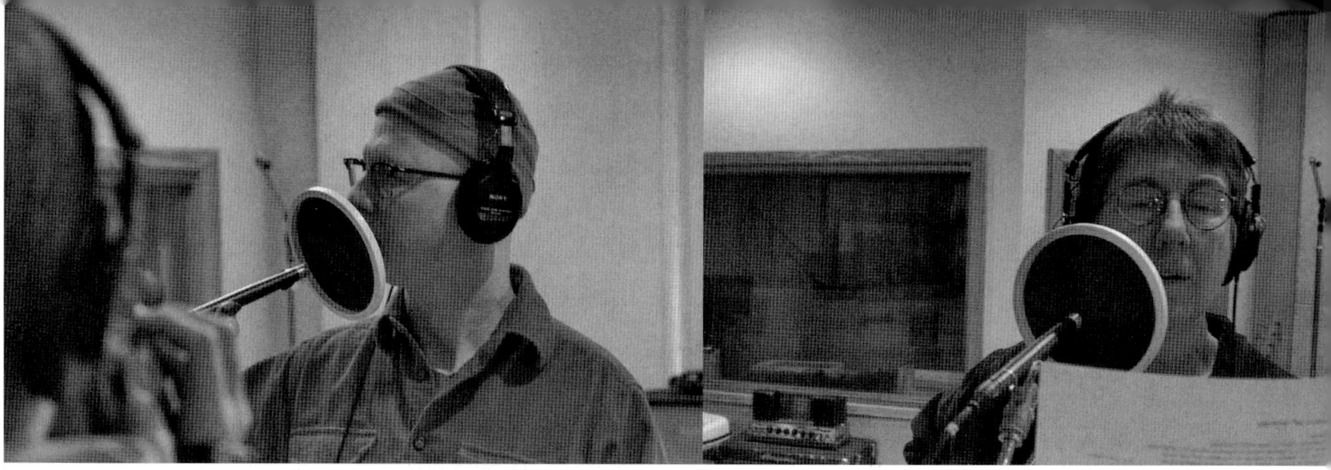

Steve and Julia recording the final narration at SoundSpace in Yellow Springs.

be the hardest part. We were juggling so much—fine cutting the picture, looking for shots that were incorrectly labeled so we could match them to their original tapes, upgrading to new computers and a new version of Final Cut Pro because the old one did not have the tools we needed to get the project completed.

And it was the holidays! As many hours as I put in during the Thanksgiving and Christmas holidays, I know John Mays and Amy Cunningham worked even harder as they recorded and mixed ambiences and foley (sound effects) for the film. It was a team effort, and I thought I had gone through the hardest part and arrived safely on the other side of it when we attended the Sundance Film Festival.

But I was wrong again.

STEVEN:

Finishing the film was utterly exhausting. Here we are, already fighting to make it to the top of the mountain we set out to climb years earlier. The last push—from August through December of 2005—we knew would take everything we had. Plus, we were starting from a state of total weariness. I guess that's the way it is with all big projects. You have to find some kind of will to keep going even though you're ready to collapse.

JULIA:

I was worried about Steve's health. He was so burned out, and he started complaining about chest pains. I was worried he'd have a heart attack.

STEVEN:

I was worried about it, too—which looking back is all part of the awful irony, that we were focused on my health instead of Julia's.

JULIA:

We were both pushing ourselves way beyond our limits. Steve got a stress test in October, to make sure he wasn't about to keel over.

STEVEN:

Another irony is, of course, that I'm noticeably younger than Julia. Our age difference hasn't ever been a big deal. In fact, if you spend some time with us, you realize that Julia is in spirit younger than me.

But it made me mad when the nurse said I wouldn't be able to outlast the treadmill. I did, and they told me my heart was in excellent shape. That small piece of info mattered hugely to my ability to get through the next three months.

KAREN:

One test of this community's effectiveness came when Julia and Steve began to show the close-to-finished-product to the families, after *Lion* was accepted into the Sundance Film Festival. Revisiting such a painful time was bound to be difficult and scary for the families, and some of the scenes did not lend themselves to easy acceptance.

STEVEN:

I was, and am, in awe of the generosity of each family after they saw the film for the first time. Each one of them, despite all the hardships of their own cancer battle, expressed concern and empathy for the other families, for how hard it had been for the other kids and families. That kind of big-heartedness just gave me such faith in humanity—in our ability to transcend our hardships. Showing the film to the families, though, was hard. The film has many upsetting moments, and different points of view and opinions in the film about what happened, what all went down and how it went down. During the screenings, members of each family talked back to the screen, even got mad at some of the stuff that was said. But to a person, each parent said they would leave it as is; that it was real, and hard, that it had to be shown. They had signed on to tell the truth, to show how complex and hard this cancer journey is, and they showed a great generosity and resolve by sticking to that decision.

DAN MISCH, Key Production Assistant:

Because part of my job required that I go through hundreds of hours of unedited footage, I feel I got to know the children and families. This was all without having ever personally met any of the families or children in the film. I cared about each of them, worried about them and grieved for them. I still do.

When I began, I never anticipated learning about life, as well as filmmaking. The families, children, and doctors in *Lion,* and Julia and Steve themselves, have taught me a lot about

The Woods and Lougheed families hanging out in the condos at Sundance.

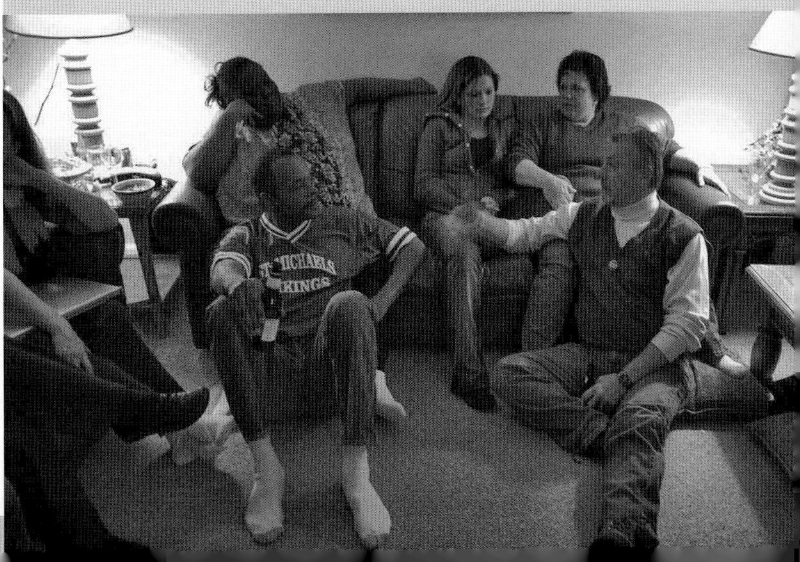

living. This film has shown me first-hand how people keep moving forward at times when it seems unimaginable to do so.

JULIA:

All hell broke loose when we got the news from Sundance. We couldn't believe our good fortune. Weeks earlier, we had joined the annual, national ritual of anxious waiting that thousands of filmmakers do every year. It's a surreal kind of process—we all send in our films, and we all wait, and we all try not to obsess or think about it.

Now because our film is four hours long, we sent it to them in the hopes that they would consider showing it once, as a special screening. We didn't even hope that they would put it in the actual festival, for instance in the *Spectrum* section or the top of the heap, the Documentary Competition.

Marietha Woods had invited us up for Thanksgiving to her new home in Massillon near Canton, Ohio. We hadn't seen her in months and were eager to show her the film. We had a wonderful time with the Woods at Thanksgiving, and stayed the night. When we got home the Friday after Thanksgiving, I was thinking how lucky we are to know that family, and that ultimately the chance to know all the families in our film matters more than getting into some big festival.

STEVEN:

Then we saw there was a message on the phone from Shari Frilot, one of the senior Sundance programmers. Immediately we were buzzing—What does it mean? What could it mean? For all we knew they had made all the acceptance calls, all the congratulations calls, and now they were doing the condolence calls.

JULIA:

We made contact, she asked what we were doing, and we explained how we were editing and just got back from showing the film to Marietha. Then she said, "Well, that's good. And you're also going to be showing the film in the documentary competition at Sundance."

STEVEN:

It was crazy. They had never shown a film that long in competition. It made for some serious logistical challenges for them.

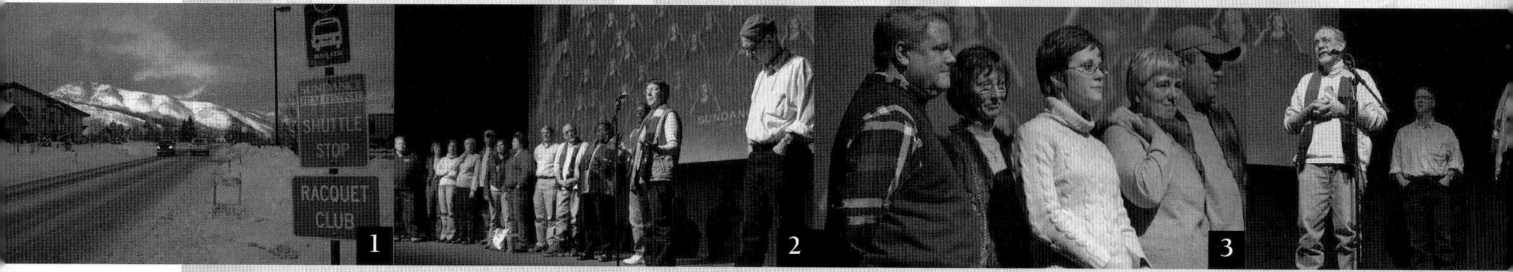

JULIA:

And it kicked our lives into complete chaos. It threw us into an overdrive we had never experienced before.

ANNE:

Those last few months, Steve, Julia, Jim Klein and I all spent a lot of time in the bungalow shaping the project into what it is today. We left a lot of blood, sweat and tears on those walls. The work of editing *A Lion in the House* was far more emotional than I had imagined it would be. I tried to keep reminding myself that it was only a film. But it wasn't.

I was dealing with real flesh-and-blood people dealing with incredibly difficult situations. I felt it deeply whenever I worked on scenes, whether it was Alex dancing with her father or Debbie crying on the phone to Adam. I was not present in the room with the families when these events actually occurred, but I can't count the number of times I've watched them struggle with diagnosis, treatment, death, and survival. Out in the bungalow, nobody remained untouched. The real challenge was to honor the children and their families by making *A Lion in the House* the best film that it could be. I hope we have done our job and done it well.

STEVEN:

From the end of November through early January, our lives were not our own. Julia was tired all the time. But when you're working almost 20 hours a day and you haven't had a day off in months, of course you're tired all the time. We were both wrecks. Also she had terrible back and neck pain, so much so that she had to start sleeping sitting up. We thought it was because of the stress and the strange beds we slept in during a long trip to New York, on the run day and night—it was far more unhealthy than we ever imagined.

JULIA:

When I got back from New York in early January, the next day I saw my doctor and got a chest x-ray. I had to deal with the increasing pain. A few days later, on Friday the 13th of January, as it turns out, my doc called and said, "There's something on the X-ray. We have to do a CAT scan."

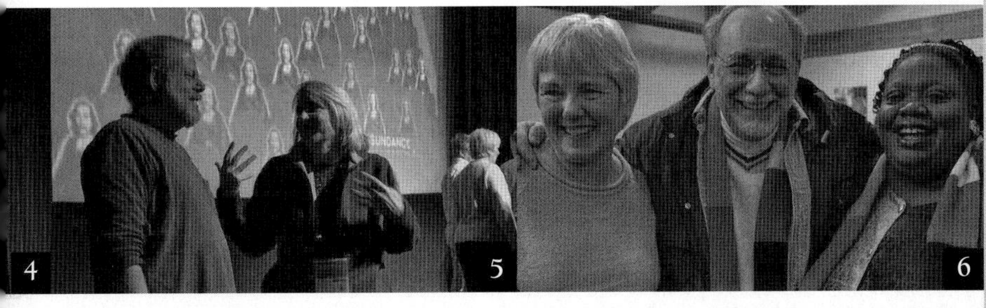
4 5 6

1. Dawn comes to Park City Utah during the 2006 Sundance Film Festival.

2. After the world premiere of A Lion in the House *at the 2006 Sundance Film Festival, the Ashcrafts, Lougheeds, Woods families, some of their doctors, Julia and Steven took to the stage in an emotional Q & A.*

3. Dale, Susan, Jennifer, Debbie & Adam during the first Q & A. While they had seen the film before the festival, the experience of watching it with an audience was powerful..

4. Dr. Arceci answering a question during the Q & A. He later said the film had exceeded his expectations.

5. Editors Jim Klein and Mary Lampson after the first screening at Sundance.

6. After the first screening, the emotional and intense conversations continued, but for many of the families and doctors in the film, it was also a reunion.

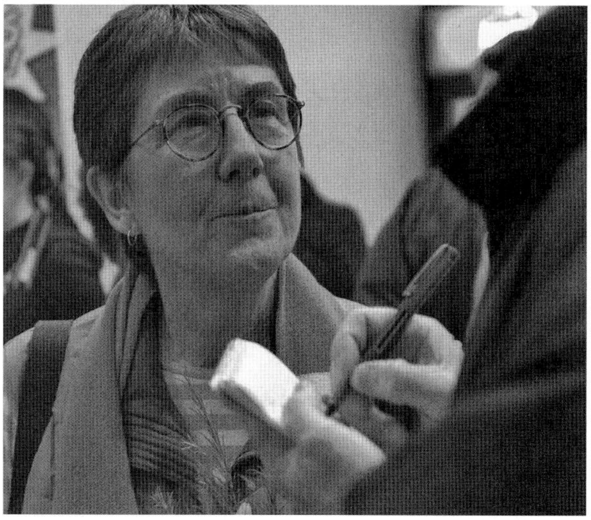

Julia put on a brave face at Sundance, but the size of the tumor pressing against her chest, coupled with the high altitude of the festival, made it difficult for her to breathe.

STEVEN:

We were just leaving that morning for Los Angeles, to present the film to the Television Critics Association winter meeting, along with Al and Regina and Dr. Arceci. Julia's doctor said we could go because it was the weekend, but as soon as she got back on Monday, she would need to get the scan.

JULIA:

In L.A., Regina and Dr. Arceci both talked to me about my health. Regina is hyper observant; she picked up right away that something wasn't right. She said I needed to go get checked.

STEVEN:

We got back on Monday morning. That afternoon Julia had the scan.

JULIA:

The next day, January 17, we went in to see our doc, Dr. Anja Shah, and she told me there was definitely a large mass in my chest. She didn't use the word "cancer," but she said it didn't look good. That day was the tenth anniversary of my daughter Lela's cancer diagnosis.

STEVEN:

The next day Julia got a biopsy, thanks to the fast work of Dr. Thomas Merle at Kettering Medical Center outside Dayton. We left for Sundance two days later.

JULIA:

When we got off the plane in Salt Lake City, I turned my phone back on and there was a message to call the doctor for the biopsy results. And there at the gate, standing next to the rows of bucket seats, with everyone pulling their roller bags past us, I heard that I had cancer—a large mass of lymphoma.

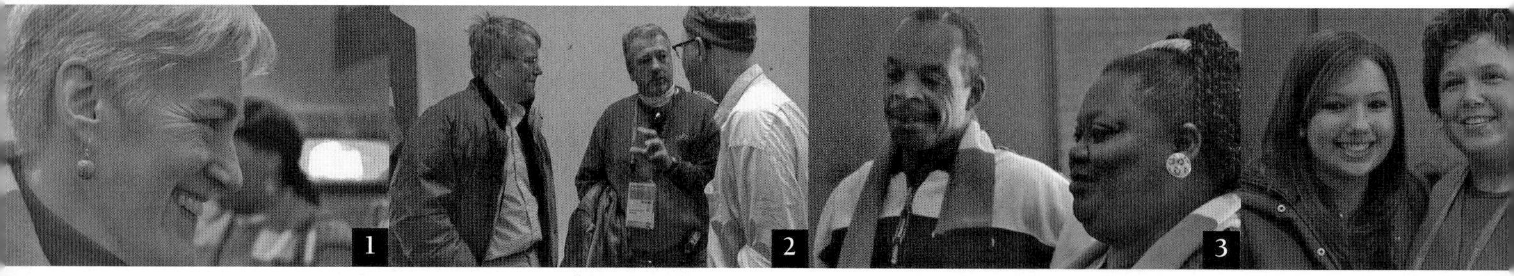

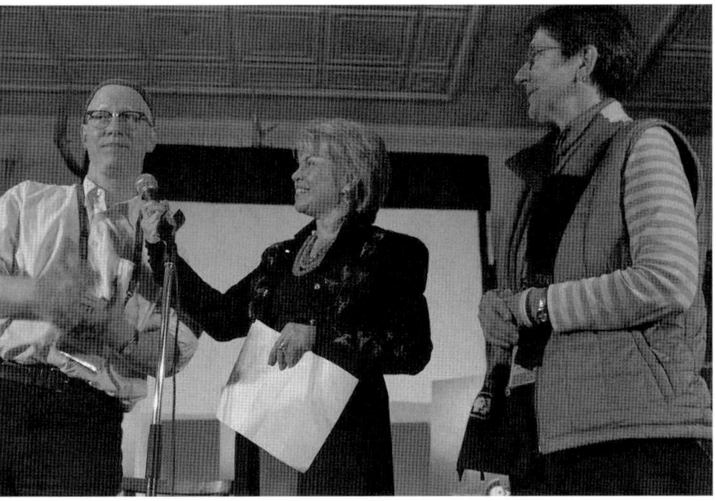

Steven & Julia are asked to say a few words by Pat Mitchell, then-President of PBS, at the PBS party at Sundance.

MELISSA:

Julia announced to a few of us that she suspected she had cancer just before Sundance. She received the certain news en route, after deplaning in Salt Lake City. When she got to the condo in Park City, she was having trouble breathing from the tumor in her chest and the high altitude, and she had to rest by the fire. Then, this take-charge director had no trouble being cared for.

Publicly, she rose to every occasion: press conferences, photos, answering audience questions after screenings. She quietly contemplated whether or not to tell people at this most public event, how, when—and decided ultimately that she must be completely honest with those who had been so honest with her.

Two nights later, after we had laughed our guts out watching the blooper reel, Julia announced her cancer. Still glowing from the outtakes, the families, crew, and friends from ITVS fell silent. Some had come to know by then, but facing it together in one energized room was new. The support grew ferociously and has sustained her since. She has not been shy about appreciating every prayer and get-well card. She has not felt sorry for herself and is open about her fears.

ANNE:

The hardest part has been getting the news of Julia's cancer. With her diagnosis coming ten years to the day that her daughter Lela was diagnosed, the timing was so ironic as to be unbelievable. It broke all of our hearts to realize that Julia and Steve had a whole new fight on their hands after working so hard to finish the film.

KAREN:

My journey with Steve and Julia began when I returned home to care for a relative with end-stage diabetes. My family and I watched and supported my Aunt Annie as she went

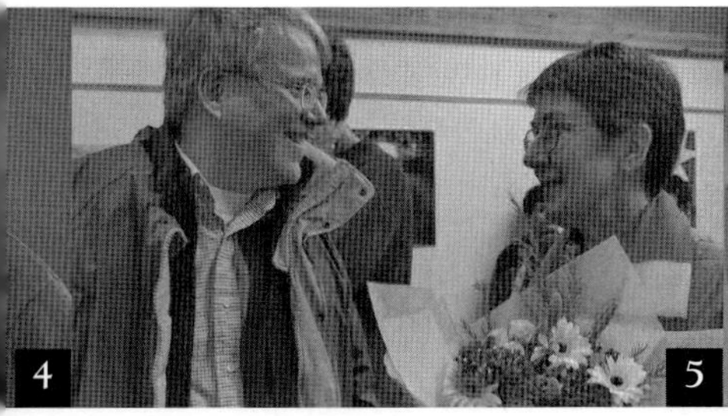

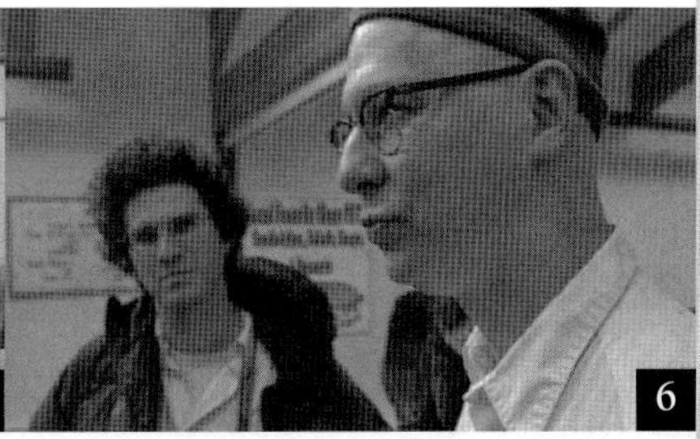

1. Susan Latton, who had spent nearly two years working on the outreach campaign for A Lion in the House*, was meeting the families and doctors in the film for the first time at Sundance. This is true for many of the editors, as well, who had lived and breathed the stories of these families for years, yet never met them in person.*

2. Dr. Paul Jubinsky, Scott Lougheed and Steven Bognar, catching up.

3. Marietha Woods and Ron Thomas discussing the film.

4. Jackie and Judy Lougheed at the world premiere. As difficult as it was to watch the film, Judy felt a need to be there.

5. Dr. Paul Jubinsky and Julia catching up.

6. Award winning director Joshua Marston (Maria Full of Grace) and his friend Steven Bognar catching up.

through the loss of one toe after another, a foot and leg, then, the other toes on the other leg. Scenes from *Lion* were like a raft in a flood. When things seemed out of control, I considered little Jen taking control by starting to count to endure the pain of a spinal tap, or Tim refusing to give up after a debacle with a feeding tube. I was prepared by the Ashcrafts for the time when my family had to discuss the living will and do-not-resuscitate order. When my precious Auntie finally passed away, I was reminded that life would go on, because it did for the Lougheeds, Woods, and Ashcrafts.

But nothing, honestly nothing, prepared me for Julia's diagnosis of cancer.

Following my Auntie's death, there was no time to grieve, no time to rest or begin to heal. *Lion* post-production went into high gear, especially following the Sundance announcement, and I began to work around the clock like everyone else. Slower than most of those I worked with, I had to acknowledge that I didn't have the ability to keep up the pace going on around me. I was becoming increasingly overwhelmed and my mistakes were many. There were few boundaries here, and I didn't have the vision or strength to establish them, especially now that my Aunt had passed and my care-taking role was gone.

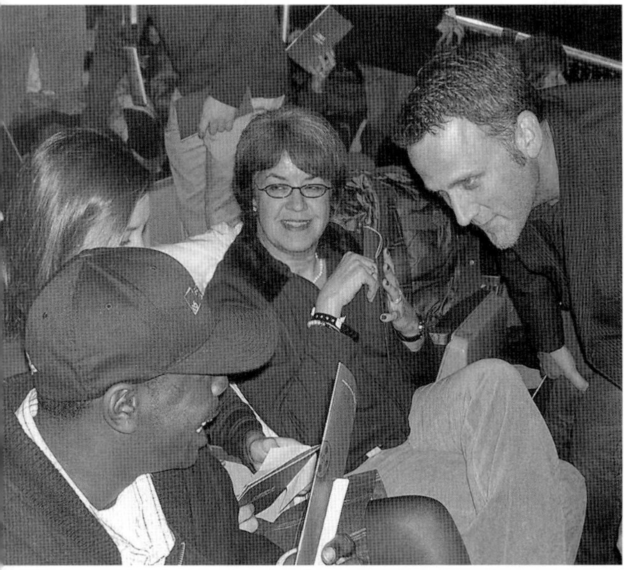

Al Fields, Jen and Beth Moone and Jim Sommers of ITVS were very happy to meet each other at the festival.

Julia and Steve, diligent proponents of excellence in filmmaking, were working 18 to 21 hour days, even on weekends, trying to meet deadlines for Sundance and for PBS. Everyone was pushing him or herself and inspiring others to stay at it and also doing crazy hours. We were so close to the finish line. I did not see the signs of Julia's illness; I guess none of us did. In many ways, Julia and Steve seemed indefatigable.

Even though Sundance was cut short for Julia and Steve, it was such a high point for the film, for outreach, but most of all for the filmmaking team, the families, docs, crew, and ITVS. We were bonded together by Julia's announcement of her cancer diagnosis.

Priorities shifted dramatically and immediately, but not before the world had a chance to see the premiere of *Lion*. The film received standing ovations, even as the family members relived their own nightmares, and the nightmare for Julia and Steve and their family was just beginning. Various team members emerged as natural leaders, and I began to experience a sense of order that made things seem more manageable even in the midst of chaos.

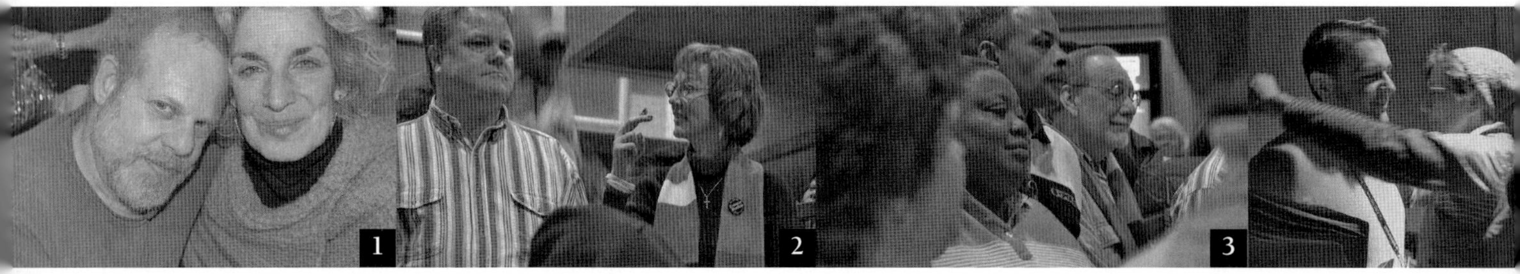

We invited people to listen to the stories of the kids, all the way through, and many did. We acknowledged that cancer is a horrible, life-changing journey, hardest on those with the fewest resources, and we need one another to get through it. People started stepping up to the plate. Compassion in action—Julia and Steve's mantra—your personal presence, positive thoughts and prayers, and doing practical things for and with families both as individuals and in community, are the ingredients that make the difference. That is the story of *Lion*.

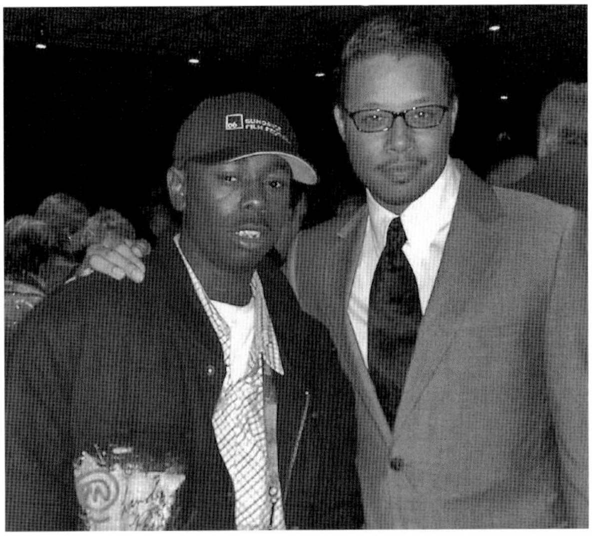

Al Fields meets Academy Award nominee for Best Actor (and Sundance jury member) Terrance Howard.

STEVEN:

We got home from Sundance on Sunday, January 22. We were admitted to the James Cancer Hospital on Monday, January 23, and did not leave for the next three weeks. The first day, we met Dr. Pierluigi Porcu, a lymphoma expert who would become Julia's trusted doctor. He looked at the results of the biopsy Julia had had in Dayton. It appeared that something had gone wrong with the pathology report, or that Julia had an exceptionally rare cancer, which was quite unlikely. Dr. Porcu ordered a new biopsy, and poor Julia had to be operated on again. A few days later, we found out the first pathology was correct, that Julia had an exceptionally rare form of lymphoma.

What happened next was among the most scary and intense things I've ever been through. With the clock ticking and the tumor growing in Julia's chest, we began a process of figuring out which treatment to do. The nature of Julia's cancer meant we couldn't do any standard, successful protocol. Whatever she chose would ultimately be a leap of faith, a gamble. We talked for hours to Dr. Porcu, who impressed us with his never seeming to be in a hurry, with the respect and responsibility he gave us.

JULIA:

He had no resistance or ego about us going to other institutions, getting second opinions. We were talking to Dr. Arceci every day, connecting us to lymphoma experts at Johns

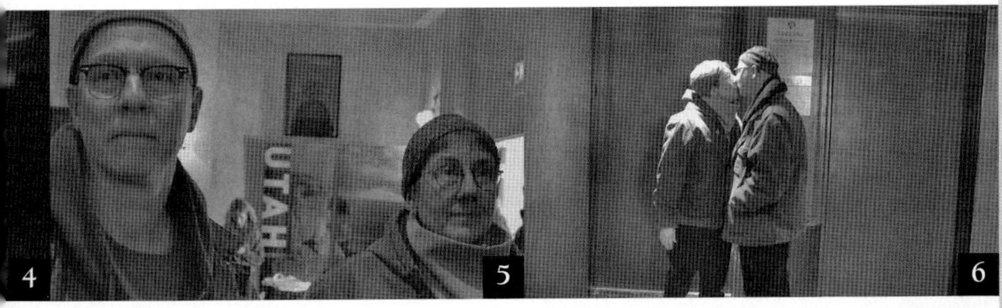

4

5

6

1. Editor Jim Klein and Diane Chiddister at the Lion *premiere dinner.*

2. Dale and Susan after the third screening at Sundance.

3. Marietha Woods, Ron Thomas and Bob Arceci during the Q & A after the third screening at Sundance.

4. Randall Cole, ITVS head of publicity, says goodbye to Julia before she heads home to face her own cancer challenge.

5. Steve and Julia leave Sundance, full of worry about the future.

6. A reassuring kiss.

Hopkins, where he now runs the Pediatric Oncology division. Jay Silver of the Intercultural Cancer Council stepped in to make contact with the oncologists he knew at M.D. Anderson in Houston. We also consulted with leading lymphoma experts at Stanford, Northwestern, the University of Nebraska, and the National Cancer Institute. Working in documentary trains you as a researcher, as an interviewer, as a note taker, as a judge of divergent viewpoints, and as a decision maker. Each of these skills were tested in us greatly, and in Lela, too. One thing we were told repeatedly was that the first treatment you use matters most. That you don't want to pick the wrong weapon, as it were, and then be one down in the fight.

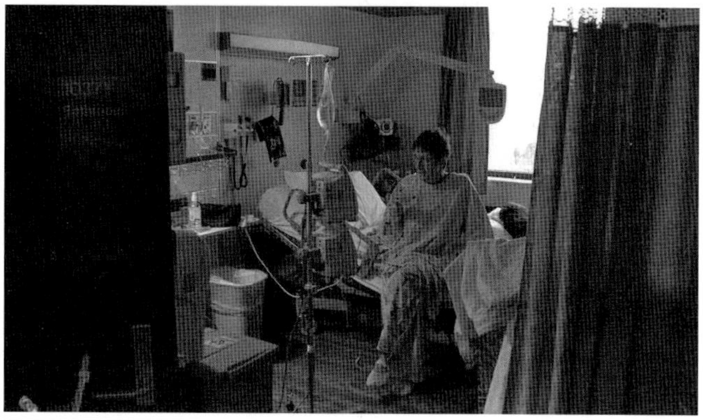

Julia, soon after first admission to the James Cancer Hospital in Columbus, Ohio. Arriving at a diagnosis took about ten tense days. Daughter, Lela, and Steve were always there, day and night.

STEVEN:

We were suddenly like the families in our film. The burden of responsibility was suddenly on us. And you know what—it was scary as hell. Lela had, post Sundance, moved back to Ohio from Chicago to be there for her mom. Lela is smarter than any of us, and it was crucial that she was there.

JULIA:

The families of *Lion* were not only a great support, they were great mentors. The years we spent with them made me less afraid, and had taught us all so much, about being proactive, being assertive, being clear.

I didn't have that much of an idea of what it is to go through cancer treatment. Which should sound funny, coming from me, with my own daughter having fought cancer, with the years spent making the film. But it's different when it's you. Which is why I wear my "cancer sucks" button.

Lela Reichert Klein and her proud mother, Julia, at Sundance. A week later, Lela would move back to Ohio to take care of Julia.

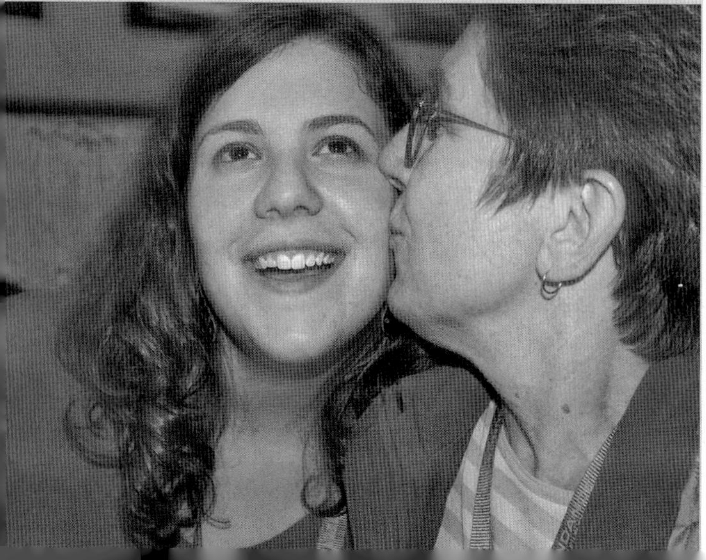

STEVEN:

We (meaning Julia, with the support of Lela and Steve) ultimately decided on a certain protocol called EPOCH, developed at the National Cancer Institute, by a team led by Dr. Wyndham Wilson. It's new, but early data show much promise. Ten days after we arrived at the James, Julia began her first round of chemo. It was awful, how she suffered. The nausea, pain and nightmares were overwhelming. But the support she got, that we all got, in those early days and even now, was an unbelievable, huge boost—it was deeply helpful, the cards, notes, thoughts, prayers, photos, gifts, music, videos and much more—it all made a huge difference to know that many people were rooting for her. Cards started showing up from all over the country. In our little town, several friends got together to create a web site (www.ysfriends.org) that gives people in need a way to state their need and friends and neighbors a way to sign up to help with meals, chores, or to get health updates.

Plus, Julia is so strong, so willful, and graced with such an indomitable spirit that she got through those hard first weeks.

About a month later, after round two of chemo, Julia went in for a series of scans, which would determine if and how well the plan was working. This was also scary, but the scans showed her tumors had shrunk dramatically, that she was exceeding expectations. She is now soldiering through the rest of her chemo rounds, buoyed by tremendous support of family, friends and community, and if all goes well she should be done with chemo by mid-summer. Then we hope to take the break that we didn't get when we finished the film.

MELISSA:

To me, *Lion*—the film and its creators, subjects and world-class crew all together—is about grace. It's about staring down the barrel of the lens at truth and finding pain, but also joy, even during moments when fate is kicking you in the butt.

When we recognize that we are all midwives to each other in the endless cycle of birth, death, and rebirth, we treat each other differently, toast each other with much more respect.

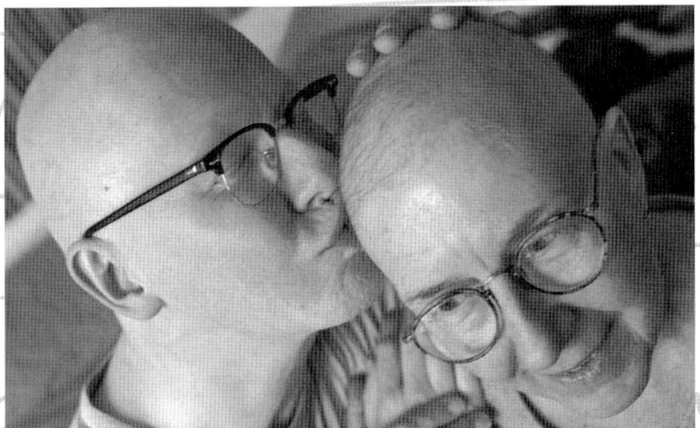

Bald Beauties: Steve and Julia in the middle of Julia's cancer fight.

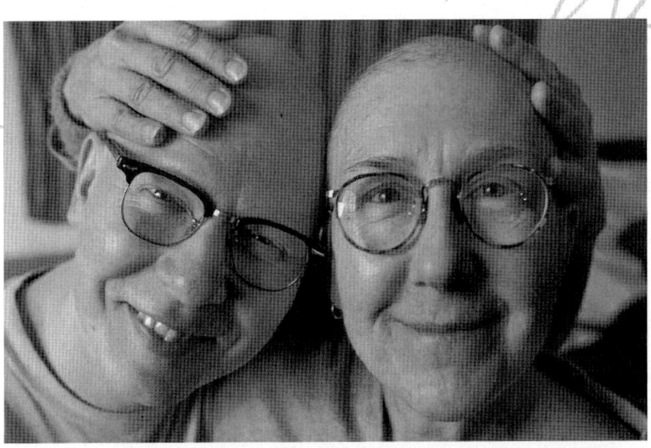

Steve and Julia, looking forward.

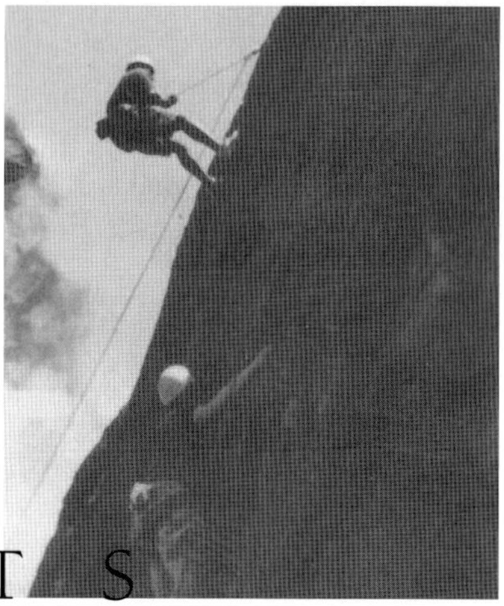

Chapter 9

Do's and Don'ts

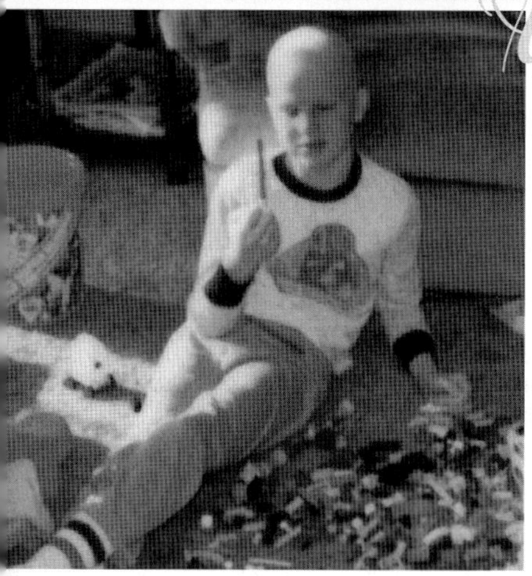

Justin, Christmas morning 1988

When a child falls ill with a catastrophic disease, the shock waves hit relatives, friends and neighbors as surely as the immediate family. Yet our instinct to lend a hand can be inhibited by awkwardness or fear of giving offense. People who appear in A Lion in the House were asked for advice on what to say and do—or not say and do—to support families coping with child's life-threatening disease. Virtually all said two things: Give the parents a break from their hospital vigil whenever possible, and always be ready to listen. That simple advice encapsulates the overriding message that families need their friends and relatives more than ever when facing a medical crisis. In their own words, here is what they suggested:

Be there! No matter what it takes, be there. No matter what is going on in your busy lifestyle, be there. Because when that person is gone, you are going to wish you had been there.—*Marietha Woods*

Have fun with the kids. Take the boys to football, take the girls to the movies. If they're in the hospital, play a board game with them.—*Al Fields*

Even if you do say the wrong thing, don't immediately pack up everything and run away. People make mistakes and say the wrong things in those situations. The worst thing you can say, "If you ever need anything, give us a call." Then that's it. When the family is in the middle of that, they're not going to say, "I need to talk to somebody." They're just too wrapped up in it.—*Adam Ashcraft*

It bothered me when people would say, "I know how you feel," but they didn't. I'd think, "You can go home with some healthy kids, and I have a sick child. So you don't know how I feel." If they had said, "I don't know how you feel, but I'm there with you," that would have been different. You just can be there if I want to talk. *—Regina Fields*

I had a hard time being around people that were complaining about things that I felt were so trivial compared to what I was going through. I really had to be careful to step back from that and think, 'I would have been that way three years ago.'*—Beth Moone*

People don't really know what to say, so they try to avoid it. They don't want to ask questions or find out. That is not the thing to do. I don't really begrudge anyone for that. It's a touchy situation, but just talking about Justin was therapy for me. *—Dale Ashcraft*

Some friends of ours stopped coming around us. They were uncomfortable. They didn't know what to do. They were worried. They were afraid of saying the wrong thing. We are all human; don't quit coming around because of that. Don't discuss their illness all the time. Treat them like any friend or neighbor.*—Debbie Kenner*

People say that, "Everything is going to be just fine," or, "Your child is going to be fine," or, "Don't worry so much." You can't just gloss it over like that. These families need to grieve and know that their child is sick. There is a real potential that some of these kids will not make it. When you say that everything is going to be fine, you don't allow families to express their fears and emotions.*—Dr. Cynthia Delaat*

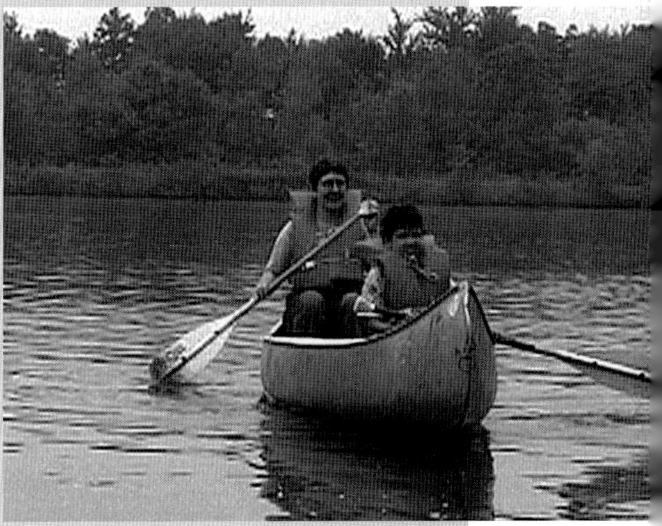

Alex canoeing with Julia. Camp is a safe place for the kids to try new things and play.

Realize that there will be good days and bad ones and changes can happen quickly. Bring in food for the families, offer to stay with their child so the parents can have a night away from the hospital. Help out with siblings that might feel left out. Assist with fund drives to help defer costs that the family might have.*—Linda Polman RN*

Help the family by giving them a break from the severely intense lifestyle that most of them will be going through—helping with the other children, running errands, etc. What they should *not* do is overwhelm the family with pity and sympathy. They should also not say that they understand what the family is going through unless they have had an identical experience.*—Dr. Vinod Balasa*

A lot of the time we see the extended family and friends show up when the child is diagnosed and come in for their first couple of treatments, but after that they do not seem to come around as much. The parents need the support every time the child comes to the hospital. Some of the treatments that these children undergo last for months to years.—*Connie Koons, RN*

Remember the child. You may have personal differences or different views or you may be angry. Do not let that get in the way of doing what is best for the child. You have to put all those differences aside and group together.—*Dr. Fred Huang*

Help the family keep their life as close to normal at home. There are siblings who need to go to basketball practice or school. Do their wash or go to the grocery for them. Be there as a listening ear. It gets scary and overwhelming emotionally and very fatiguing.—*Dr. Cynthia Delaat*

Do not forget about the siblings. Many times people feel sorry for the child with the cancer and buy them lots of gifts and forget about how this is also affecting the siblings. During times like this, the siblings need just as much attention as the sick child.—*Connie Koons, RN*

What should they *not* do or say? That they can imagine what the family of the patient is going through. They really have no idea.—*Dr. Paul Jubinsky*

You can't try to change what is going on. Be there, be supportive, not directive. Don't confuse the issues. Listen. Listen more, talk less. I think the most important thing is: Don't become somebody different.—*Dr. Robert Arceci*

Julia's List of Practical Advice

As the mother of a childhood cancer survivor and the beneficiary of eight years close observation of the families in A Lion in the House, *filmmaker Julia Reichert developed the following set of suggestions for those who wish to do something useful for patients and their families.*

How to help...

When you say, "Don't hesitate to ask me for anything," keep repeating that offer.
Rake the family's leaves.
Weed their garden.
Take their car to the shop.
Pick up groceries.
Cook a meal. Better yet, agree to cook a meal every week.

Find out what the patient really wants to eat and make that.
Offer to sit with a sick child and read or watch a movie.
Offer to take the siblings on a walk or window-shopping.
Find out what the sibs want to do, and do that.

How not to help ...

Don't avoid the family. If you're nervous about visiting, send a card.
If you want to help and don't know what to do, ask someone close to the family. (It's smart for a family to assign someone besides the parents to be the go-to person for information and updates.)
Don't wear the parents out.
Don't drain their energy by asking them to tell the same things again and again.
Don't bring up hard topics unless they want to go there.

Good gifts ...

Soft pajamas. Flannel (good for air-conditioned hospitals); button up the front (easier for IV lines and exams)
Silk flowers (Real ones are often prohibited).
Soft blanket.
Squishy pillow. Or, for a child, a pillow or pillowcase with an age-appropriate character.
Easy to put-on slippers for cold hospital floors.
Cards, funny cards especially.
Pictures of things the patient loves.
Books of jokes or cartoons.
Notes or drawings from classmates and church friends. Cancer treatment goes on for months, and often more than one year, so send another card, or another batch of drawings.

Chapter 10

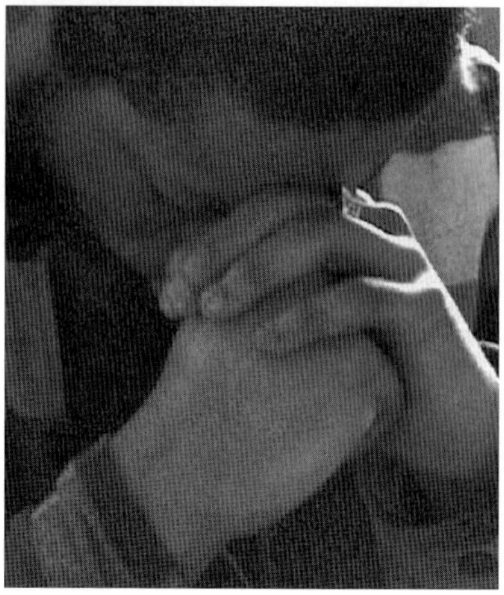

How
TO GET HELP
HOW TO GIVE HELP

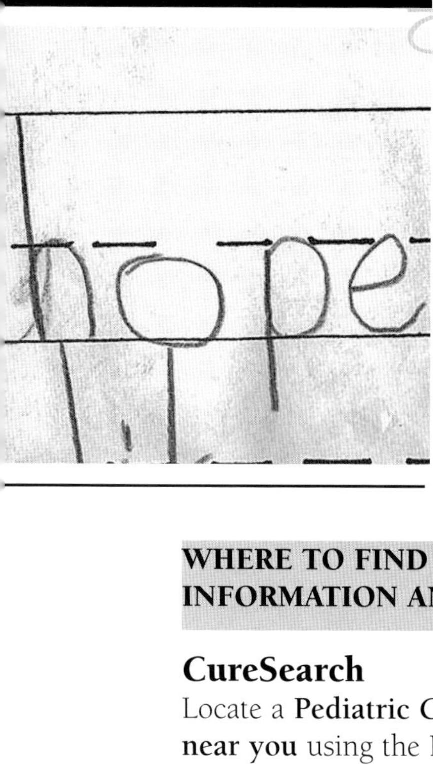

From the beginning, everyone involved in A Lion in the House *committed to using the project to educate and encourage cancer patients and their families, as well as the thousands of others engaged in battling the disease.*

Critical to that battle are the services provided by the following distinguished organizations, which contributed support, expertise and advice during production of A Lion in the House*. The Lance Armstrong Foundation and Centers for Disease Control also lent financial support. These organizations collectively represent a wealth of state-of-the-art knowledge organized to serve the needs of people touched by cancer. Likewise, they offer multiple opportunities to raise money for research, to lobby for governmental action, and to volunteer to offer direct help to families. Full description and contact information for each organization begins on page 139.*

WHERE TO FIND TREATMENT, INFORMATION AND CLINICAL TRIALS

CureSearch

Locate a **Pediatric Cancer Treatment Facility near you** using the **Directory of COG member institutions.**

www.curesearch.org/resources/

See web site below and click on:

CureSearch Clinical Trials Information Service for a clinical trials matching service, which allows users to identify available trials in hospitals nationwide.

Medical information customized to a child's diagnosis, age and treatment phase.

For Parents/Families or For Patients to access the **Resource Directory.**

www.curesearch.org

"What was my reaction to finding out Jen had cancer? Oh, I was just devastated."
—Beth Moone (Jen's Mother)

National Cancer Institute

Search the **National Cancer Institute's (NCI) Physician Data Query (PDQ), a comprehensive cancer database**, for: **Childhood cancer information and clinical trials** www.cancer.gov/cancertopics/types/childhoodcancers

Childhood cancer treatment summaries

www.cancer.gov/cancertopics/types/childhoodcancers

Childhood Cancer Resources

ctep.cancer.gov/resources/child.html

Children's Cause for Cancer Advocacy

Search for **new treatments for childhood cancer and clinical trials**.

www.childrenscause.org/resources/finding_clinical_trials.shtml

Children's Cancer Association

Click on **Kid's Cancer Pages**, which is recognized by the NCI as "the most comprehensive resource guide available to children and families suffering with cancer."

www.childrenscancerassociation.org

Hope Street Kids

Search the **Online Parent Guide for key questions to ask at diagnosis and in seeking treatment and clinical trials.**

www.hopestreetkids.org/parent_guide/diagnosis.php

Learn the do's and don'ts of effective childhood advocacy.

www.hopestreetkids.org/advocacy_education/dos_and_donts.php

Candlelighters

For information on **Complimentary & Alternative Medicine, Clinical Trials, and Late Effects**, click on **Treatment**.

www.candlelighters.org

KEY RESOURCES FOR EMOTIONAL ISSUES FACING TEENS AND CHILDREN WITH CANCER

Planet Cancer

On-line support, insights, and information for older teens/young adults and a clearinghouse of information on regional gatherings of support and networking are available.

www.planetcancer.org

"Why do you think I drink and stuff? To keep my mind off stuff. When I drink on certain weekends and I go out, have fun with my friends, I'm not thinking about stuff. I'm not down. I'm not sitting at home crying. I'm having fun, at least I think. Or I'm trying to make myself have fun. When I'm not doing that, I'm thinking about stuff and I get depressed."
—Tim Woods

Starlight Starbright Children's Foundation

Click on **Programs** to find **"Coping With Chemo Webisodes" written by teens, Starbright World, an online community for Teens, and Explorer Series CD ROMs.**

www.starlight.org

SuperSibs!

Advocacy and support services for siblings.

www.supersibs.org

"It's hard for a twelve-year-old to understand. Justin always had to take first for everything. I was very jealous."
—Jennifer Ashcraft (Justin's sister)

Teens Living with Cancer

This **online support group for teens** is available in English and Spanish.

www.teenslivingwithcancer.org

The Wellness Community

Click on **Group Loop, an online support group for teens.**

www.thewellnesscommunity.org

American Cancer Society

Look Good...Feel Better is both an online and free support program for teenage cancer patients 13 to 17 years old that helps them cope with the appearance-related side effects of cancer treatment.

www.2bMe.org

"The only thing that was so hard to me is that I had to learn don't worry about what other people think, because even though I look different, I know I wasn't different. I was the same old person."—Al Fields

Candlelighters

Click on **Kids** and explore web sites, books and song resources. Click on **Advocacy** to learn about the **Childhood Cancer Awareness Tree**.
www.candlelighters.org

Make-A-Wish Foundation of America

Grants wishes to children with life-threatening medical conditions.
www.wish.org

BACK TO SCHOOL SUPPORT

The Leukemia & Lymphoma Society

For **The Trish Greene Back to School Program for Children with Cancer**, click on **School and Youth Programs**. The program, **Welcome Back: Facilitating the Return to School for Children with Cancer**, and **a free booklet**, are available by calling
800-955-4572.
Learn about **Pennies for Patients and other fundraising programs for kids**.
www.schoolandyouth.org/school/Controller

Candlelighters

Request a free book: *Educating the Child with Cancer: A Guide for Parents and Teachers.*
www.candlelighters.org

Starlight Starbright Children's Foundation

A Back to School MTV Style Video and Videos with Attitude
www.starlight.org

American Cancer Society

Kids can support their peers fighting cancer by participating in **fundraising activities like Relay for Life.**
www.cancer.org

Hope Street Kids

Learn about the **Kids Walk for Kids with Cancer Annual Fundraising and Advocacy Event**. www.hopestreetkids.org

SCHOLARSHIPS AND CAMPS

Children's Oncology Camping Association International

www.coca-intl.org

Ulman Cancer Fund for Young Adults

College Scholarship Listings
www.ulmanfund.org.

American Cancer Society

College Scholarships for Cancer Survivors and Camps for young cancer patients, many at low or no cost to the camper.
www.cancer.org or call 800-ACS-2345

SURVIVOR RESOURCES

CureSearch

Directory of Long-Term Follow-Up Guidelines
www.survivorshipguidelines.org
Late Effects Directory of Services (and Long-Term Follow-Up Clinics)
www.childrensoncologygroup.org

Centers for Disease Control and Prevention

The Survivor Alert Project (in partnership with A LION IN THE HOUSE) seeks to educate young adult survivors of childhood cancer about their risks for long-term effects from their treatment.
www.survivoralert.com
The National Action Plan for Cancer Survivorship: Advancing Public Health Strategies, is a resource book developed in partnership with the Lance Armstrong Foundation.
www.cdc.gov/cancer/survivorship/index.htm

National Cancer Institute

The Office of Cancer Survivorship
www.survivorship.cancer.gov

Lance Armstrong Foundation

Livestrong Survivorship Notebook helps cancer survivors organize and guide their cancer experience. Order a free **LIVESTRONG™** Survivorship Notebook.
www.livestrong.org/notebook

Livestrong SurvivorCare provides individual counseling, aid with legal, financial and/or insurance issues and matching to clinical trials. See the web site or call toll free 866-235-7205 to speak to professional oncology social workers. **LAF Community Program** awards grants to nonprofit organizations to serve people living with cancer.
www.livestrong.org/communityprogram

Planet Cancer

Online support, insights, and information for older teens/young adults and a clearinghouse of information on regional gatherings of support and networking are available.
www.planetcancer.org

National Children's Cancer Society

The NCCS Beyond the Cure program hosts Teleconferences and Survivorship conferences on a variety of issues and concerns experienced by survivors and their families after completion of treatment for childhood cancer. **For a Listing of Long-Term Follow-Up Clinics that follow COG guidelines,** click on **Survivorship**, then click on **Resources. To Build a Personal Late Effects Assessment**, click on **Personal Profile**, and click on **Register to Build A Late Effects Assessment.**
www.beyondthecure.org

Fertile Hope

Call **1-888-994-HOPE** or look for the following resources:
Cancer and Fertility: A Guide for Youth Adults
Childhood Cancer and Fertility: A Guide for Parents
Cancer and Fertility Resource Guide
Sharing Hope Financial Assistance Program
www.fertilehope.org/download_brochures.cfm

Gilda's Club Worldwide

Noogieland, a play area for children, and Weekly Programming that address the social and emotional needs of cancer survivors and their families and friends, are available through Gilda's Club.
www.gildasclub.org

National Coalition for Cancer Survivorship

Learn more about survivorship resources:
The Cancer Survivor Toolbox
The Guide to Minority Cancer Survivorship Program
CanSearch First Steps: Step-by-step guide to online cancer resources
www.canceradvocacy.org/resources/

Patient-Centered Guides

Click on **Childhood Cancer Survivors** for excerpts and info on the resource book, *Childhood Cancer Survivors*.
www.patientcenters.com

Children's Cause for Cancer Advocacy

Rise to Action Survivorship Workshops educate survivors about the importance of knowing their diagnosis and treatment history and how to access health information, and empowers young survivors with advocacy skills. Ask about **Translating Our Voices into Action: Challenges in Pediatric Cancer Advocacy**—national advocacy workshops for parents and survivors—by calling (301) 562-2765 or by Email: questions@childrenscause.org
www.childrenscause.org

Ulman Cancer Fund for Young Adults

Learn more about the **Patient Advocate/Navigator Program, the Speaker's Bureau, and the Survivor's and Loved Ones Network**, among other resources.
Find information on an **Education and Prevention Curriculum for Middle School, High School and College**.
www.ulmanfund.org

National Cancer Survivor's Day

Locate a **Listing of Survivor Events** that occur on the first weekend in June all around the country and for a **National Cancer Survivor's Day Planning Kit.**
www.ncsdf.org

PALLIATIVE, END-OF-LIFE, AND BEREAVEMENT CARE

National Hospice and Palliative Care Organization

The NHPCO Directory offers a search for a hospice, pediatric palliative care or bereavement, and end-of-life provider and/or coalition programs in your community in Spanish or English.
www.nhpco.org/custom/directory/main.cfm

PartnershipForParents.org is a national website for parents of seriously ill children and for families grieving the loss of a child.
www.PartnershipForParents.org

The Children's Project on Palliative/Hospice Services has resources for health professionals available through www.nhpco.org/marketplace: Caring for Kids: How to Develop a Home-Based Support Program for Children and Adolescents with Life-Threatening Conditions (CD only), Education and Training Curriculum for Pediatric Palliative Care, Compendium of Pediatric Palliative Care

Children's Hospice International

Worldwide Database of Programs caring for children with life-threatening conditions and their families. To find a location in your community:
www.chionline.org/resources/locate.phtml

Seven demonstration projects provide a continuum of care through diagnosis, cure and bereavement.
www.chionline.org/programs/programs.phtml

National Coalition for Cancer Survivorship

Access the **Comprehensive Guide on Palliative Care & Symptom Management** by clicking on **Survivorship Issues**.
www.canceradvocacy.org

Oncology Nursing Society

Patients and caregivers learn **information about managing common symptoms secondary to cancer and its therapies**.
CancerSymptoms.org

Health Ministries Association

Locate **National offices of faith groups or religious denominations** that have an active interest in programs related to health ministry.
www.hmassoc.org/faithgrouplinks

The "Find a Church" search can lead you to local churches and potential connections with those who minister to families facing the illness/loss of a child.

National Center of Medical Home Initiatives

Find **Tools and information for families and providers on palliative care.**
www.medicalhomeinfo.org/resources/palliative.html

National Cancer Institute

Learn more about the **Institute of Medicine Report/Book on Childhood Cancer:** *When Children Die*
www.iom.edu

RESOURCES TO REDUCE AND ELIMINATE CANCER HEALTH DIPARITES

Centers for Disease Control and Prevention

Link to the President's Cancer Panel publications:

- "Living Beyond Cancer: Finding a New Balance"
- "Voices of a Broken System: Real People, Real Problems"

www.cdc.gov/cancer

Center to Reduce Cancer Health Disparities at the N.C.I.

Patient Navigator Programs have trained, culturally sensitive healthcare workers who help individuals address patient-access barriers.

The Community Networks Program launches community-based participatory education, training, and research among racial/ethnic minorities and underserved populations.

The Special Populations Networks promote cancer awareness, conducts cancer control research, initiates cancer control activities, and promotes the career development of minority junior biomedical and behavioral researchers.
http://crchd.nci.nih.gov/initiatives

Intercultural Cancer Council

The **Biennial Symposium on Cancer, Minorities and the Medically Underserved** brings together those who represent all aspects and perspectives of cancer, with the leadership and front-line personnel from the affected communities, to explore issues, find solutions, and make recommendations.

iccnetwork.org

ICC Regional Network Leadership members connect you with local contacts and organizations that can speak on issues of cancer health disparities.

iccnetwork.org/who/regionalnetworkleadership.htm

"Children/Adolescents and Cancer" is a fact sheet that covers research on disparities in child cancer care and outcomes.

iccnetwork.org/cancerfacts/cfs9.htm

Children's Defense Fund

The **CDF SHOUT Program (Student Health Outreach Project)** is a student-run program that seeks to expand outreach and enroll uninsured children in the Children's Health Insurance Program (CHIP) or Medicaid.

The National Observance of **Children's Sabbath** on the third Weekend in October mobilizes the interfaith community to address serious problems facing children and poor families. Children's Sabbath Manuals are available.

The annual Samuel Dewitt Proctor Institute for Child Advocacy Ministry Conference, where ministers, seminarians, educators, lay leaders, and other people of faith who work with and for children gather at the former Alex Haley Farm to address serious problems facing children and poor families. For more info, call (800) CDF-1200 or go to the web site.

www.childrensdefense.org

The Cancer Information Service

The CIS Partnership Program works with non-profit, private and government organizations to overcome educational, financial, and cultural or language barriers.

http://cis.nci.nih.gov/community/community.html

Padres Contra El Cáncer

PADRES services are focused in the Los Angeles area; however, they do **offer support and referrals by phone to families seeking assistance** in larger metropolitan areas in the United States and parts of Mexico and Central America.

www.iamhope.org or www.yosoyesperanza.org

Patient Advocates Foundation

Advocates around insurance issues.

Find info on **African American Outreach** listed under Resources.

Bilingual Services are available for all services offered by this organization.

www.patientadvocate.org

National Center of Medical Home Initiatives

Compassionate and culturally competent care resources are available for children and youth with special health care needs.

www.medicalhomeinfo.org/tools/compassion.html

Advocacy and spokesperson tips and background materials are listed for families and practitioners on issues of special-needs children.

www.medicalhomeinfo.org/health/advocacy.html

Find out about events and activities happening in your state that will help improve access to medical homes for children and youth with special health care needs.

www.medicalhomeinfo.org/states/index.html

Public Television Station Outreach

Learn more about the A LION IN THE HOUSE series, the outreach campaign, the filmmakers and resources, including disparities.

www.itvs.org/outreach/lioninthehouse

Contact your local public television station's outreach staff by clicking on **Outreach Directory.**

www.nationaloutreach.org

EDUCATIONAL AND PROFESSIONAL DEVELOPMENT

Association of Oncology Social Workers

The AOSW site's publication page provides links for new resources and publications, several specific to pediatric cancers:
www.aosw.org/publications/publications.html

Association of Pediatric Oncology Nurses

The Association of Pediatric Oncology Nurses publishes **selected patient/family resource materials.**
www.apon.org

CancerCare

Learn more about **Cancer*Care* Connect:** Telephone Education Workshops.
www.cancercare.org

Health Ministries Association

CEU's for nurses, clergy and chaplains, approved by their professional associations are available. The easy-to-follow directions for completing the module and receiving the certificate are available at the site.
www.hmassoc.org/continuing_education.html

The Leukemia & Lymphoma Society

Access **Pediatric Cancer Educational Series—free teleconferences** with childhood cancer experts by calling 800-955-4572.
www.lls.org

National Association of Social Workers

The NASW and CancerCare have teamed up to create **an online course called "Understanding Cancer: The Social Worker's Role."**
www.naswwebed.org/
The NASW and the Children's Cause for Cancer Advocacy have partnered to develop **a web-based educational tool for social workers** to learn about childhood cancer survivorship and strategies for working with survivors.
www.socialworkers.org

National Cancer Institute

Review the **"NCI Health Information Tip Sheet for Writers: Childhood Cancers."**
www.cancer.gov/newscenter/tip-sheet-childhood-cancers

National Center of Medical Home Initiatives

Find **Tools and Training Materials** to assess and implement medical homes.
www.medicalhomeinfo.org/tools/providerindex.html

National Children's Cancer Society

Learn more about the **NCCS Beyond the Cure program Teleconferences.**
www.beyondthecure.org

HOTLINES

American Cancer Society

(800) ACS-2345
Cancer Information Specialists are available 24 hours a day/seven days a week/365 days a year. Translation services are also available. **Patient Navigators** can link you with programs and resources in your community.

CancerCare

(800) 813-HOPE
Social Workers provide assistance in navigating the cancer journey and in developing individualized plans to manage day-to-day concerns. Learn what **financial assistance** is available.

Caring Connections

(800) 658-8898
The **HelpLine** offers support with **end-of-life issues.**

Fertile Hope

(888) 994-HOPE
Provides support in facing **cancer-related problems with infertility.**

The Leukemia & Lymphoma Society

(800) 955-4572
Master's level Social Workers, Nurses, and Health Educators are available Monday through Friday, 9 a.m. to 6 p.m. ET.

Supplementary financial assistance is available to patients in significant financial need. Learn how to apply at www.lls.org.

National Cancer Institute

(800) 4-CANCER (422-6237).
Cancer Information Specialists answer calls in English or Spanish.

National Children's Cancer Society

(800) 5-FAMILY (532-6459).
Gives **financial and in-kind assistance**, advocacy, support services, and education.

Patient Advocates Foundation

(800) 532-5274
Provides **assistance in resolving insurance, job retention and/or debt crisis matters** relative to a patient's diagnosis, with translation services available.
Co-Pay Relief Program—www.co-pays.org

About the Organizations

Public Television Station Outreach
(www.itvs.org/outreach/lioninthehouse)
Independent Television Service (ITVS), co-producer of A LION IN THE HOUSE, and the Lance Armstrong Foundation provided grants of as much as $10,000 to local public television stations that aired A LION IN THE HOUSE to pay for educational activities in their own communities.
Phone: (415) 356-8383 • Fax: (415) 356-8391
Email: itvs@itvs.org
Independent Television Service
501 York Street
San Francisco, CA 94110

American Cancer Society
(www.cancer.org)
The American Cancer Society is the nationwide community-based voluntary health organization dedicated to eliminating cancer as a major health problem by preventing cancer, saving lives, and diminishing suffering from cancer through research, education, advocacy and service.
Phone: (1-800) ACS-2345
TTY: (1-866) 228-4327
1825B Kramer Lane, Suite 200
Austin, TX 78758

Association of Oncology Social Workers
(www.aosw.org)
Oncology social workers provide a wide range of services directly to persons with cancer and their families, including counseling, support, education, and resource identification. As advocates, AOSW and its members are dedicated to increasing awareness about the social, emotional, educational and spiritual needs of cancer patients through conferences, research, writing, workshops and lectures.
Phone: (215) 599-6093 • Fax: (215) 545-8107
Email: info@aosw.org
100 North 20th St., 4th Floor
Philadelphia, PA 19103

Centers for Disease Control and Prevention
(www.cdc.gov/cancer/)
The Centers for Disease Control and Prevention (CDC) is a leader in nationwide cancer prevention and control, working with national organizations, state, territorial and tribal health agencies and other key groups to develop, implement and promote effective cancer prevention and cancer control plans. The plan charts a course for how the public health community can more effectively and comprehensively address cancer survivorship and focus on improving the quality of life for survivors.
Phone: 1-800 CDC-INFO (232-4636)
Fax: (770) 488-4760 • TTY: 1 (888) 232-6348
Email: cdcinfo@cdc.gov
National Center for Chronic Disease Prevention and Health Promotion
Division of Cancer Prevention and Control
Mail Stop K-64, 4770 Buford Highway, NE
Atlanta, GA 30341-3717

Children's Cause for Cancer Advocacy
(www.childrenscause.org)
The Children's Cause for Cancer Advocacy (CCCA) is a non-profit organization that works as a national catalyst to stimulate drug discovery and development for childhood cancers, to expand resources for research and treatment and to address the needs and concerns of survivors.

Phone: (301) 562-2765 • Fax: (301) 565-9670
Email: questions@childrenscause.org
1010 Wayne Avenue, Suite 770
Silver Springs, MD 20910

CureSearch
(www.curesearch.org)
CureSearch represents the combined efforts of the Children's Oncology Group (COG) and the National Childhood Cancer Foundation (NCCF), two organizations united by a common goal: reaching the day when every child with cancer can be guaranteed a cure.
Phone: (800) 458-6223
Email: info@curesearch.org
National Childhood Cancer Foundation
4600 East West Highway, Suite 600
Bethesda, MD 20814-3457
Children's Oncology Group (COG)
Research Operations Center
440 E. Huntington Drive
P.O. Box 60012
Arcadia, CA 91066-6012

Gilda's Club Worldwide
(www.gildasclub.org)
Gilda's Club Worldwide is a free cancer support community for men, women and children with any type of cancer and their family and friends. Membership is offered free of charge to people at any stage of their experience with cancer.
Phone: (888) GILDA-4-U
Fax: (917) 305-0549
Email: info@gildasclub.org
322 Eighth Avenue, Suite 1402
New York, NY 10001

Health Ministries Association
(www.hmassoc.org)
Health Ministries Association (HMA) is an interfaith membership organization, serving the people who serve the Faith Health Ministry Movement. The mission of HMA is to encourage, support and develop whole-person ministries leading to the integration of faith and health.
Phone: (800) 280-9919 • (770) 640-9955
Fax: (770) 640-1095
295 W. Crossville Rd., Suite 130
Roswell GA 30075

Hope Street Kids
(www.hopestreetkids.org)
Hope Street Kids (HSK) is an initiative of the Cancer Research and Prevention Foundation. HSK was founded by Randy Walker and Congresswoman Deborah Pryce in memory of their nine-year-old daughter, Caroline. Its mission is to eliminate childhood cancer through cutting-edge research, advocacy and education.
Phone: (800) 227-2732 • (703) 836-4412
Fax: (703) 836-4413
1600 Duke Street, Suite 500
Alexandria, VA 22314

Intercultural Cancer Council
(www.iccnetwork.org)
The Intercultural Cancer Council (ICC) promotes policies, programs, partnerships and research to eliminate the unequal burden of cancer among racial and ethnic minorities and medically underserved populations in the United States and its associated territories. Baylor College of Medicine assumes fiscal and organizational management for the Intercultural Cancer Council and provides the Council with a national office and website.
Phone: (713) 798-4617 • Fax: (713) 798-6222
Email: info@iccnetwork.org
6655 Travis, Suite 322
Houston, TX 77030-1312

The Lance Armstrong Foundation
(www.livestrong.org)
The Lance Armstrong Foundation (LAF) believes that in the battle with cancer, unity is strength, knowledge is power and attitude is everything. From the moment of diagnosis, the Foundation provides the practical information and tools. People living with cancer need to live strong.
Phone: (512) 236-8820 • Fax: (512) 236-8482
Lance Armstrong Foundation
P. O. Box 161150
Austin, TX 78716-1150

The Leukemia & Lymphoma Society
(www.lls.org)
The Leukemia and Lymphoma Society (LLS), headquartered in White Plains, New York, is dedicated to funding blood cancer research and

providing education and patient services. The Society's mission is to cure leukemia, lymphoma, Hodgkin's disease and myeloma, and to improve the quality of life of patients and their families.
Phone: (914) 949-5213 • 1-800-955-4572
Fax: (914) 949-6691
1311 Mamaroneck Ave.
White Plains, NY 10605

National Association of Social Workers
(www.socialworkers.org)
(www.helpstartshere.org)
The National Association of Social Workers is an organization of professional social workers with the mission to promote, develop and protect the practice of social work, while enhancing the well-being of individuals, families and communities through its policy work and advocacy.
Phone: (202) 408-8600
750 First Street, NE Suite 700
Washington, DC 20002-4241

National Black Nurses Association, Inc.
(www.nbna.org)
The National Black Nurses Association (NBNA) mission is to provide a forum for collective action by African American nurses to investigate, define and determine what the health care needs of African Americans are and to implement change, to make available to African Americans and other minorities health care commensurate with that of the larger society.
Phone: (301) 589-3200 • (800) 575-6298
Fax: (301) 589-3223
Email: NBNA@erols.com
8630 Fenton Street, Suite 330
Silver Spring, MD 20910-3803

The National Cancer Institute
(www.cancer.gov)
The National Cancer Institute (NCI) is the largest institute within the National Institutes of Health (NIH). NCI provides extramural funding to support research, training, health information dissemination, and other programs with respect to the etiology, diagnosis, prevention, and treatment of cancer, rehabilitation from cancer, and the continuing care of cancer patients and their families. NCI's Cancer Information Service (CIS), the Center to Reduce Cancer Health Disparities, and the Division of Cancer Control and Population Sciences, Office of Survivorship are helping to advise the *A Lion in the House* outreach campaign.

American Academy of Pediatrics/National Center of Medical Home Initiatives
(www.aap.org)
(www.medicalhomeinfo.org)
The American Academy of Pediatrics (AAP) is committed to the attainment of optimal physical, mental and social health and well being for all infants, children, adolescents and young adults. The AAP also houses the National Center of Medical Home Initiatives for Children with Special Needs that promotes a model of care for special needs children called "medical home." A pediatric clinician works in partnership with the family/patient to assure that the medical and non-medical needs of the patient are met. The care plan combines palliative care and life prolonging care for children and youth living with life-threatening or terminal conditions and their families. The Medical Home Initiative is supported by HRSA and its Bureau of Maternal and Child Health and provides the potential to extend supportive services to childhood cancer patients and survivors.
Phone: (847) 434-4000 • Fax: (847) 228-7035
The National Center of Medical Home Initiatives
141 Northwest Point Blvd.
Elk Grove Village, IL 60007

National Hospice and Palliative Care Organization
(www.nhpco.org)
The National Hospice and Palliative Care Organization (NHPCO) is committed to improving end-of-life care and expanding access to hospice care with the goal of profoundly enhancing quality of life for people dying in America and their loved ones. The NHPCO advocates for the terminally ill and their families. It also develops public and professional educational programs and materials to enhance understanding and availability of hospice and palliative care, convenes frequent meetings and symposia on emerging issues, provides technical informational resources to its membership, conducts research, monitors Congressional and regulatory

activities, and works closely with other organizations that share an interest in end of life care.
Phone: (703) 837-1500 • Fax: (703) 837-1233
Email: nhpco_info@nhpco.org
1700 Diagonal Road, Suite 625
Alexandria, VA 22314

Oncology Nursing Society/Association of Pediatric Oncology Nurses
(www.ons.org)
(www.apon.org)
The Oncology Nursing Society (ONS) is a professional organization for registered nurses and other healthcare providers whose mission is to promote excellence in oncology nursing and quality cancer care. Their sister organization, the *Association of Pediatric Oncology Nurses* (APON) is the leading professional organization for registered nurses caring for children and adolescents with cancer and their families.
Phone: (847) 375-4724 • Fax: (877) 734-8755
Email: info@apon.org
The Oncology Nursing Society
4700 W. Lake Ave.
Glenview, IL 60025

Padres Contra El Cáncer
(www.iamhope.org)
(www.yosoyesperanza.org)
Padres Contra El Cáncer is a non-profit organization committed to improving the quality of life for Latino children with cancer and their families through support services which include case management, family educational programs, crisis intervention, support groups, economic assistance and quality of life events. All Padres activities and services, while oriented to the Latino community, serve childhood cancer patients from all races and ethnic origins. Services are focused in the Los Angeles area; however, they do offer support and referrals by phone to families seeking assistance in larger metropolitan areas in the United States and parts of Mexico and Central America.
Phone: (800) 269-4186 • (323) 850-7901
Fax: (323) 850-7914
3479 Cahuenga Blvd. W
Los Angeles, CA 90068

OTHER RESOURCES:

CancerCare
(www.cancercare.org)
Cancer*Care* is a national non-profit organization that provides free professional support services to anyone affected by cancer: people with cancer, caregivers, children, loved ones, and the bereaved.
Phone: (212) 712-8400 • (800) 813-4673
Fax: (212) 712-8495
275 7th Ave.
New york City, NY 10001

Candlelighters
(www.candlelighters.org)
Candlelighters Childhood Cancer Foundation is committed to its mission of providing support, education and advocacy for children and adolescents with cancer, survivors of childhood/adolescent cancer, their families and the professionals who care for them.
Phone: (301) 962-3520 • (800) 366-2223
Fax: (301) 962-3521
P.O. Box 498
Kensington, MD 20895

Children's Cancer Association
(www.childrenscancerassociation.org)
The Children's Cancer Association (CCA), a nonprofit organization, was established in memory of five-year-old Alexandra Ellis, who died after a two-year battle with cancer. CCA offers award-winning programs, along with information, advocacy and support that help enrich the quality of life for seriously ill children and their families.
Phone: 503-244-3141 • Fax: 503-892-192
7524 SW Macadam, Suite B
Portland, OR 97219

Children's Defense Fund
(www.childrensdefense.org)
The mission of the Children's Defense Fund is to Leave No Child Behind and to ensure every child has a Healthy Start, a Head Start, a Fair Start, a Safe Start, and a Moral Start in life and successful passage to adulthood with the help of caring families and communities.
Phone: (202) 628-8787

Phone: (800) CDF-1200 (800-233-1200)
Fax: (202) 662-3580
E-mail: cdfinfo@childrensdefense.org
25 E Street, N.W.
Washington, D.C. 20001

Children's Hospice International
(www.chionline.org)
Children's Hospice International (CHI), a nonprofit organization, was founded in 1983 to promote hospice support through pediatric care facilities, encourage the inclusion of children in existing and developing hospice, palliative, and home care programs.
Phone: 703-684-0330 • Fax: 703-684-022
901 North Pitt Street, Suite 230
Alexandria, VA 22314

Children's Oncology Camping Association International
(www.coca-intl.org)
Children's Oncology Camping Association International, C.O.C.A., is an international assembly of people providing camping programs for children with cancer. Many member camps serve a broad range of special needs populations, but all share the common thread of working with pediatric oncology patients.
Phone: (515) 243-6239
1221 Center Street, Suite 12
De Moines, IA 50309

Fertile Hope
(www.fertilehope.org)
Fertile Hope is a nonprofit organization dedicated to helping cancer patients faced with infertility.
Phone: 1-888-994-HOPE
P.O. Box 624
New York, NY 10014

The Make-A-Wish Foundation of America
(www.wish.org)
We grant the wishes of children with life threatening medical conditions to enrich the human experiencees with hope, strength, and joy.
Phone: (800) 722-WISH (9474)
Fax: 602-279-0855
3550 N. Central Ave., Suite 300
Phoenix, AZ 85012

National Cancer Survivor's Day
(www.ncsdf.org)
National Cancer Survivor's Day is held annually in hundreds of communities throughout the world on the first Sunday in June. It is a symbolic event to demonstrate that life after a cancer diagnosis can be a reality.
Phone: (615) 794-3006 • Fax: (615) 794-0179
Email: info@ncsdf.org
P.O. Box 682285
Franklin, TN 37068-2285

The National Children's Cancer Society
(www.beyondthecure.org)
(www.nationalchildrenscancersociety.com)
The mission of The National Children's Cancer Society (NCCS) is to improve the quality of life for children with cancer by promoting children's health through financial and in-kind assistance, advocacy, support services, and education.
Phone: (314) 241-1600 • (1-800) 5-FAMILY
Fax: 314-241-1996
1015 Locust, Suite 600
St. Louis, MO 63101

National Coalition for Cancer Survivorship
(www.canceradvocacy.org)
The National Coalition for Cancer Survivorship is a survivor-led cancer advocacy organization and a highly respected authentic voice at the federal level, advocating for quality cancer care for all Americans and empowering cancer survivors.
Phone: (301) 650-9127 • (877) 622-7937
Fax: (301) 565-9670
1010 Wayne Ave., Suite 770
Silver Springs, MD 20910

Patient Advocates Foundation
(www.patientadvocate.org)
Patient Advocate Foundation is a national nonprofit organization that seeks to safeguard patients through effective mediation assuring access to care, maintenance of employment and preservation of their financial stability.
Phone: (757) 873-6668 • (800) 532-5274
Fax: (757) 873-8999
8700 Thimble Shoals Blvd., Suite 200
Newport News, VA 23606

Planet Cancer
(www.planetcancer.org)
Planet Cancer is a community of young adults with cancer. "It's a place to share insights, explore our fears, laugh, or even give the finger to cancer with others who just plain get it. We don't deny the dark side of illness and death here. But we also firmly believe that laughter and light can turn up in the strangest places."
Phone: (512) 452-9010 • Fax: (512) 451-3110
2710 Cedar Street
Austin, TX 78705

Starlight Starbright Children's Foundation
(www.starlight.org)
Starlight Starbright Children's Foundation is a non-profit organization dedicated to making a world of difference for seriously ill children and their families.
Phone: (310) 479-1212 • (800) 315-2580
Fax: (310) 479-1235
1850 Sawtelle Blvd., Suite 450
Los Angeles, CA 90025

SuperSibs!
(www.supersibs.org)
Our goal is to reach out to the brothers and sisters of over 12,600 children in the U.S. and Canada who are diagnosed with cancer each year. Through our work, these siblings will feel valued, validated, heard, supported and delighted as recipients of SuperSibs! services and as participants in SuperSibs! activities.
Phone: (847) 705-1132 • (866) 444-7427
(cell) (847) 778-4451
Fax: (847) 776-7084
4300 Lincoln Ave., Suite I
Rolling Meadows, IL 60008

Ulman Cancer Fund for Young Adults
(www.ulmanfund.org)
To provide support programs, education and resources, free of charge, to benefit young adults, their families and friends, who are affected by cancer, and to promote awareness and prevention of cancer.
Phone: (888) 393-FUND • (410) 964-0202

The Wellness Community
(www.thewellnesscommunity.org)
The Wellness Community (TWC) is an international non-profit organization dedicated to providing support, education and hope for all people affected by cancer, at no cost.
Phone: (202) 659-9709
Fax: (202) 659-9301
919 18th St., NW, Suite 54
Washington, DC 20006

Youth Service America
(www.ysa.org)
Youth Service America is a resource center that partners with thousands of organizations to increase the quality and quantity of volunteer opportunities for young people, ages five through twenty-five, to serve locally, nationally, and globally. YSA's mission is to strengthen the effectiveness, sustainability, and scale of the youth service and service-learning fields.
Phone: 202-296-2992 • Fax: 202-296-4030
1101 15th Street, Suite 200
Washington, DC 20005